1

Tears in My Gumbo

In my 40+ years of clinical practice as a Licensed Clinical Social Worker, I have not found such an impressive and valuable resource as this book. It is written with sensitivity and expertise. Nadine presents a unique book with compelling vignettes and concrete approaches to caregiving while providing an empathetic and informed guide supporting those who provide compassionate care.

> *JoKatherine Holliman Page, MSW, LCSW*
> *Denver, Colorado*

This book is a great read! It takes our understanding of caregiving to a unique place. This author weaves together a complex tapestry of her experiences as a family caregiver and professional caregiver. She is one of those rare and inherently talented storytellers. This is a wonderful, joyful and hopeful work that will speak to people of all ages and persuasions. Cornish's wealth of deep experience as a caregiver shines through with spiritual strength and integrity. This is a must read for those involved in eldercare as well as for anyone who knows or cares for someone providing care. Take the time to savor this special gumbo.

> *Sue Bozinovski, Ph.D.*
> *Facilitator, Denver–Boulder Professional Advancement*
> *Certificate in Gerontology*

I LOVED the stories. Nadine is a warm, rich, deep and lyrical writer. She drew me in with the framing of the stories and her language. My experience was one of curiosity, wonder, compassion, appreciation, joy, sadness, and love. She rang the bell on all of my emotions! I LOVE, LOVE, LOVE the gumbo metaphor. Each chapter is rich with a personal, deeply touching and therefore, connecting story.

Sam Trenka
Navigator Coaching and Consulting

I thought reading this was going to be hard for me because I envisioned reading facts about a life that I was going to dread. But it was refreshing. It flowed, inspired and gave guidance with simple directives about what caregivers have to encounter and endure.

Roslyn Cary, Caregiver
Exton, PA

I have read through this manuscript three times now, and was never able to read it in one sitting because of the emotions the piece evokes from my life personally. I will tell you I have never read anything that touched me the way this writing has touched me. This is a beautiful tribute to caregivers any and everywhere.

Earl X Wright
Retiree, Buckley WA

The "recipe" is a must for those on the cusp of caregiving. I found myself reflecting on my seven years of caregiving for a 105-year young great aunt. This is a necessary handbook in the field of caregiving.

> *Carlotta Walls LaNier*
> *Author of* A Mighty Long Way
> *Caregiver*

I planned on reading this slowly over the course of a week, but I couldn't put it down and read it in one sitting. This is a book that should be in every household, every physician and clinic waiting room, every home health and hospice agency, and shared with every home palliative care and hospice nurse. This book will surely become tattered as it will be passed on from generation to generation.

> *Eileen Thomas, PhD*
> *RN Nursing Professor*
> *Community Public Health*
> *University of Colorado*

This is a masterpiece, a Jewel of Love and personal triumph in the face of adversity and uncertainty! As a Family Medicine Physician, this book opened my mind and my heart again to see how one can turn obstacles and road blocks into a creative success. The ability to care for another human life and spirit, is beyond incredible. *Tears in my Gumbo* is the secret sauce to caregiving.

> *NaNotchka M. Chumley, D.O., M.P.H*
> *Family Medicine Physician*
> *Los Angeles, CA*

Tears in My Gumbo is a delightful read that whets your appetite for more stories by Nadine Cornish. From her personal and professional experiences as a caregiver, she dishes up soul-full stories about caregivers and care receivers. Nadine highlights the key ingredients needed if we are to care well and be well over the course of the caregiving journey. *Tears in My Gumbo* is truly a recipe for success. Savor every word and allow the stories to feed your soul. No doubt, you will feel blessed after reading the book—as do I.

> *Jane W. Barton, MTS, MASM, CSA*
> *Author of Caregiving for the GENIUS*
> *Cardinal, LLC*
> *Caregiving Ambassador for AARP Colorado*

TEARS

IN MY GUMBO

TEARS
IN MY GUMBO

BOOK ONE

THE CAREGIVER'S RECIPE
FOR RESILIENCE

NADINE ROBERTS CORNISH

Books may be purchased in bulk by contacting
the publisher at:
CaregiversGuardian@gmail.com

Cover Photo: Nadine Roberts Cornish
Cover Design: Liana Moisescu
Interior Design: WESType Publishing Services, Inc.
Publisher: Caregivers Guardian Publishing House
Editors: Cynthia Schoen Editing Services
John Maling, Editing by John

First Edition
Library of Congress Catalog Number: 2016914991

ISBN paperback: 978-0-9980691-0-4
eISBN: 978-0-9980691-1-1
Audio: 978-0-9980691-2-8

1. Caregiving   2. Aging   3. Healthcare   4. Self-Care
5. Elder Care   6. Self-Help   7. Spirituality/Religion

Printed in the USA

To my mother,

Elizabeth Vivian Catherine St. Cyr Roberts,
you were my first and greatest teacher. You
exemplified dignity, grace, class and self-respect.

Thank you for continuing to watch over me.

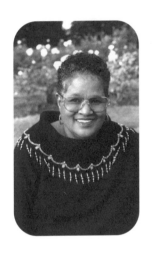

Contents

Foreword

Life is full of twists and turns. The unexpected is the norm. We know this but the role of the caregiver is a part that no one can be prepared to experience. You can know it is coming. You can think that you are ready, yet feelings of overwhelm and powerlessness can rush in without warning. Most of us have a deep desire to be present and do the right thing for the people we love when they are in need. However, we do not come encoded with a manual on caregiving.

At this moment, the baby boomers are coming of age as the caregivers of the generation before us. Most of us are ill equipped. We are also in denial that we are old enough to become the "parents of our parents." Some of us step up and take a stand for the people we love. Others withdraw and run as fast as they can from the pain and the process of the caregiver's journey. No matter how you handle it, there is no way to predict the process or the duration of this call to action.

I did not grow up with gumbo as a regular part of a diet dictated by family. It was something that was brought into my life well into my twenties. I was not aware of how much time, energy, love and skill it took to prepare this glorious dish. Today, that understanding makes me begin to comprehend that making this dish is the perfect metaphor for the life and times of a caregiver.

I have known Nadine Cornish for several years. She went through my Freedom Coach training and often spoke about how much she loved her work and had a calling to share what she had learned with the masses. I knew she was a person of excellence and commitment. I didn't know, until reading this book, what time, energy, commitment and compassion she has invested into this courageous service to others.

This book, *Tears in My Gumbo,* is a gift. Nadine does a masterful job of sharing her personal, professional and revelatory stories. The stories are of real people that she has counseled and supported in moments of crisis and change. My heart opened as I read the story of a love so deep that it transcended illness, mental deficiencies and death. Nadine invites us into the experience of the caregiver *and* the one being cared for. She gently reminds us that we must be prepared because the need to care for another can come in an instant. We, the readers, are asked to take her recipe and get ready for the feast of our lives. She guides us through tender preparations, the gentle sauté, gracious seasoning, and heavy boiling pots, with dexterity. This feast is our tribute, our daily bread, and sometimes the last supper for our loved ones.

I had many personal responses reading this book, including wondering what care I will need when I move toward the end of my life experience. I certainly wish I had been given this book when my mother, at 86 years old, could no longer function on her own. We realized when she was in her seventies that we needed to get her paperwork in order. What we didn't understand is that when I took on the role as her power of attorney I would be put into positions that were challenging at best. I had to make decisions for the woman who raised me and supported me my whole life.

I wanted to show up powerfully. I wanted to care for her. However, as her care became more complex and time consuming, and as she became at times combative, I felt clueless and anxious on many occasions. I clearly did not have the ingredients I needed to create and deliver a powerful "meal" of support.

Tears in My Gumbo is for anyone who is already a caregiver, becoming a caregiver or knows a caregiver who can use support. I sincerely hope that you will give yourself the gift of this book and share it with others. I have a feeling that readers will want to gift this book to many people and for a long time to come.

Let this beautiful book guide you in the process of loving and caring for others. Why not learn to make "caregiving" gumbo before you need to serve it?

Cynthia James
Author, Coach, Speaker

Introduction

Tears in My Gumbo has been eight years in the making. I thank my mother for being the inspiration and I thank God for giving me the assignment to serve, support, work with and honor family caregivers.

I often say that this is not a path that I chose. This path chose me. On some days I wanted to quit, give up or run and hide because sometimes the task seemed too hard. What I came to learn is your calling in life is not your choice. It is your duty—your charge—the reason you were placed on this earth. Working with and supporting caregivers has become my charge and I am honored to be of service.

This compilation of short stories includes my story of caregiving for my mother and grandmother and stories about a handful of the family caregivers whom I have had the honor of working with and serving. I have been granted permission to share their stories, with names and identifying markers changed to preserve their privacy. Their courage, tenacity and strength in the face of difficult odds continue to inspire and enthrall me. In turn, this collection is intended to galvanize caregivers and those who care about them. This book is based upon my own personal and professional experiences, and my conclusions may not be applicable in all circumstances.

Throughout the book I have used my family recipe for Louisiana Seafood Gumbo as a metaphor for the creation of caregiver resilience. Gumbo is central to the New Orleans culture where I was born and raised. Gumbo is much more than a soup and way better than a stew. It represents everything that is unique and special about my large and loud family, the beautiful essence of my mother, the spicy and strong presence of my grandmother, the power and depth of my grandfather, Edmond St. Cyr, and all the lines of people I came from stretching back to Africa, infused with French and Native American flare. Gumbo is a dish that is communal. It nourishes and it sustains.

Caregivers operate in the confluence of love and loss when they take on the care of their beloved. They need something as bold and nurturing as a recipe for gumbo to sustain them in their work, to create resilience when they feel like collapsing under the weight of their task and uncertainties.

Caregiver resilience is possible. With resilience the caregiver can keep at their task, making adjustments along the way like a seasoned chef. With guidance they can do more than sustain themselves. They can achieve a spiritual state which is both a victory and a blessing.

Each story illustrates the major ingredients needed to create the supreme dish of caregiver resilience. The conclusion of each chapter, a recipe card of essential ingredients, provides a recap of tips, instructions and the most essential elements for the recipe.

Of course a recipe is more than just a list of ingredients. It is also a series of instructions for the steps one must take in combining those ingredients. Therefore, as each caregiver's story is told, the stage of caregiving they are moving through is also noted. Just as Elizabeth Kubler Ross enabled those going through grief to understand that grief is a non-linear process with various stages (denial, anger, bargaining, depression and acceptance), this book will help caregivers become aware of the journey they are undertaking, the stages they will visit perhaps more than once, and the spiritual attainment which is possible at the culmination of this assignment.

I refer to them as the **five steps of conscious caregiving**. I began using this phrase as I started to see a distinction among the family caregivers I worked with and as I assessed my own experience as a caregiver. I would see the same patterns over and over again in every caregiving situation. I would meet caregivers who were conscious and those who were on automatic pilot. The distinction between conscious caregiving and caregiving in a reactive manner is an important one. A conscious caregiver is rooted in the experience of agape love and the sheer humanity of caring for a loved one. They take on their role with intention. They are proactive and invested, not simply going through the motions. They reach out and ask for help. They recognize the need to research, and they understand the necessity of becoming an advocate. The feeling of being a victim may be where a caregiver starts. However, the goal is to move out of that unempowered stance and become victorious.

Over time, and after studying many of my client cases, I've identified the five steps of caregiving as **helplessness, recognition, process, acceptance** and **surrender**. These stories exemplify the process a caregiver goes through as they take on their task, make the necessary preparations, commit to seeing it through, seek assistance, accept that they cannot control the course of their loved one's illness, and ultimately, achieve spiritual growth through surrender. These steps enable the caregiver to move from victim to victorious. I realize not every caregiving situation will follow the steps I have described here, but I believe many will.

Upon learning of their loved one's illness or disability, caregivers may feel **helplessness**, shock, disbelief and even resentment of the circumstances which have occurred. One day they wake up and their life has changed forever due to a catastrophe, stroke, or life threatening diagnosis received by a loved one. For others, a slow and gradual process of caregiving takes place, yet when the day arrives when their loved one requires greater care, it can be daunting. The prospective caregiver will naturally experience denial, confusion and uncertainty about what to do next or where to turn. During this step, feelings of anger and fear may surface as they grapple with the reality of the situation.

The second step is **recognition** of what is happening to the loved one. The present reality is still a fog and the role of caregiver has been temporarily accepted with some hesitation and doubt. The caregiver begins to realize decisions must be made regarding what they are willing and able to do. The novice caregiver begins to recognize a new reality is impacting their life, and they must start making life changing decisions which will not only impact their loved one but also themselves. Often during this phase, the caregiver realizes they don't know what they don't know.

Consultation, research, and understanding of the illness fortify the caregiver as they gear up and embrace their role. But still, they are not yet in action as inertia and uncertainty persist. This phase is cyclic as the caregiver begins to question their ability, question their knowledge, and even question their willingness to take on the daunting role of being the primary caregiver for their loved one.

To move out of this circular motion, which often feels like victimhood, the caregiver must begin to take action. This signifies the third step as the caregiver starts to reach out, seek help and begin the **process** of conscious caregiving. It is during this step when decisions are made to determine how the family can best support the loved one, whether there is a need to hire a professional caregiver or seek out long term care options. At this point financial and legal actions are commonly addressed. During the process step, the caregiver may request outside help, continue to gather information, establish their own expertise, enter into partnership with the medical team, and put a caregiving team together. Step three includes embracing the caregiving role, utilizing a team approach, expressing gratitude to everyone in the caregiving circle, and tapping deeper into their spiritual source.

The fourth step in the caregiving journey is **acceptance**, which begins by releasing the need to control circumstances and outcomes. The caregiver starts to realize that despite their most valiant efforts, the trajectory of their loved one's illness cannot be changed. The caregiver gains insight and begins to understand the change that must occur, occurs within them. For example, when an Alzheimer's patient no longer recognizes their caregiver, the idea of accepting what cannot be changed and simply being present in the moment becomes a viable option.

In reaching the fifth and final step of the caregiving process, the conscious caregiver learns to **surrender**. The caregiver begins to understand that they are responsible, yet not in control. Caregiving forces one, like few other things in life, to give in, to let go. For those of us blessed to know and be in relationship with our Higher Source, that is how we surrender. We let go and let God. We accept we are not in control, and allow "Thy will be done." Hopefully the caregiver will come to rest in surrender. In the stance of surrender, paradoxically, they can reach victory.

I have come to realize **acceptance** is what we do on a mental level. **Surrender** is about what we do on a soul or emotional level.

As the caregiver surrenders to their loved one's inevitable transition, and eventually their absence, they may begin to feel gratitude for all that has been given and received in the process of caring for their loved one. With guidance, the caregiver can treasure the honor of their role and begin to cherish the remarkable spiritual invitation of *Anam Cara*, a Celtic term meaning Carer of the Soul. In Ireland, professional caregivers, doctors, nurses and priests were revered for centuries for their role as caregivers to those transitioning. I've expanded this concept to include the family caregiver who is the carer of the body and the soul during the caregiving journey. I've met many caregivers who don't know the term but operate in the spirit of this beautiful concept.

The one distinct commonality that emerges over and over again in each of the stories is the basis and foundation for the act of caregiving. That commonality is simple humanity and love. Love is the secret sauce in all the recipes of caregiving and the healing source for our lives, for our world. Love is the driving force which compels a caregiver to keep giving and doing, even when others may believe there is nothing left to serve.

No caregiver should attempt to travel this journey alone. It is important for caregivers to identify resources—care managers, coaches, consultants, professional caregivers and home health agencies—who are available to assist them. Knowing you don't have to walk this journey alone makes the journey sustainable, and will be a substantial factor in maintaining sanity and stability.

The purpose of this book is to inform, encourage and inspire the caregiver and those who love the caregiver. No matter what difficulties a caregiver faces, their mission is God-inspired and ordained. This realization will carry them through the toughest and most challenging times.

This book is as much for those who care about the caregiver as it is for the caregiver. These stories illustrate what it really means to be a caregiver, with many of those challenges depicted. My hope is the champions of caregivers, their loved ones and friends, will join the caregiver in some capacity, perhaps as a sous chef, head cook, line cook or even dish washer. The point is caregivers need tangible, hands-on support and encouragement in any way others are able to provide that support.

Finally, in addition to this book being a cathartic experience for the reader, there are also sprinklings of smiles and chuckles tucked inside because there is no resilience without laughter.

recipe card

The Five Steps of Conscious Caregiving

1. **Helplessness**—The caregiver may experience shock, disbelief, denial, uncertainty, confusion, fear and even resentment at a task which appears daunting.
2. **Recognition**—The role of caregiver has been temporarily accepted with hesitation and doubt. The caregiver begins to make decisions which will impact their loved one and also themselves.
3. **Process**—The caregiver starts to reach out, seek help and begin the process of conscious caregiving. They embrace the caregiving role, use a team approach, express gratitude, and tap deeper into their spiritual source.
4. **Acceptance**—The caregiver starts to realize that the trajectory of their loved one's illness cannot be changed. They see they are not in control.
5. **Surrender**—Give in—let go—let God. We recognize we are not in control and allow "Thy will be done."

chapter one

Tears

For so long unwelcomed, I now embrace
the transformative power of each drop.

My journey as a caregiver had come to an end. I was exhausted to the core and clueless about what life post-caregiving would look like. I had many ideas about how I would pick up the life I had left behind as a Social Marketing Consultant creating public health education campaigns, but as I thought about returning to my old life, I would be engulfed in a fog.

Six months prior to her death, my mother, Elizabeth St. Cyr Roberts, had been diagnosed with Stage IV Breast Cancer. I was incredulous. My mom had been under the constant care of many doctors. She was hospitalized seven times that very year. How in God's name could she have breast cancer? I was beside myself with the pain and weight of this reality. It felt so incredibly unfair. Even though I had been the caregiver for my mother for over twelve years, I was once again experiencing the resistance of shock and denial.

Had not my mother been through enough?
Wasn't a large, pituitary brain tumor enough?
If not that, then surely a massive stroke had to be enough?

Right side paralysis?
Aphasia?
What about Hepatitis C, contracted through blood
     transfusions?
Diabetes?
High Blood Pressure?
Congestive Heart Failure?
Mild Dementia?

All of these were my mom's actual diagnoses and some-how she found the grace, strength and dignity to handle and manage them. But this—this Stage IV Breast Cancer—she didn't have a fighting chance with this. She was battle weary and didn't have any fight left in her. Once again I had found myself circling back to the stage of **helplessness**. But this time there was a difference. I had earned the spiritual grace during the previous years of conscious caregiving to receive a blessing along with the shock.

As I grabbed my hair and screamed in anguish over this bitter injustice, I heard a small voice. The voice told me, "Calm down. The cancer isn't for your mom. It's for you, to learn from."

"What? What do you mean, the cancer is for me?" The voice clearly said I would need to understand cancer in order to do the work I was assigned to do. "What work?" I asked in desperation.

"The Assignment, your work with family caregivers."

"Are you kidding me? I want to run as far away from caregiving as I can."

Who was it that was speaking to me? God? Was God so plainly and clearly talking to me?

Well, if it was Him, I needed to test Him. If He really meant what He was saying, if the cancer was for me to learn from and not for my mom, then we needed to make a deal.

My mom would not and could not suffer from this cancer. She would not become emaciated by it and it would not wreak havoc on her the way I had seen it devastate others in our family. I knew I was not supposed to bargain with God, but at the time we were in the final stages and I needed assurance. I made my peace with God and prepared myself for what lay ahead, entering the stage of **recognition** yet again.

My brothers came out to visit. We got second opinions. Radiation and chemotherapy weren't options, and surgery ultimately wasn't recommended. Neither Mom's heart nor her spirit was strong enough to handle those treatments. To cheer her up, we planned a magnificent 71st birthday celebration for Mom in beautiful Estes Park, Colorado. Due to a cancellation, we were able to rent the highly sought after reunion cabin. It is a lovely, spacious cabin with a huge great room and amazing fireplace. It had fifteen bedrooms and could accommodate up to sixty of us, all under one roof. The back wall was an entire sheet of glass looking out onto the majestic Rocky Mountain State Park.

On a glorious October weekend, sixty-two family members came from all over the country to shower Mom with love. We have a huge family, but the fact that so many people came with only six weeks' notice is a testament to the beauty of my mother's soul. My mom had the face of an angel. At times I would look at her and see a beautiful Hawaiian with full cheeks, and other times I'd see a serene Native American with a steady gaze. A girl from New Orleans, she embodied the African, French and Native American mixture so common to the people and food of that region.

As I placed photographs of her on the stone mantle, I noticed her sweet apple-cheeked smile when she was just a young girl smitten by her first love. Her face filled out over time, expressing the generosity she radiated as a middle aged woman. When her hair turned salt and pepper around her face, the generosity moved toward square-jawed wisdom. Through all the years, love and generosity permeated her being. I realized then, my mother had always been gorgeous, kind and full of love, but she had also evolved gradually into the wise woman I cherished.

On the day of arrival, and shortly after check in time, we had scheduled a professional photo shoot to capture the entire family. Due to so many folks getting lost or taking the scenic route and arriving late, we didn't meet at the appointed time or location for the shoot. Unfortunately for the photographers, they came to the cabin at the same time that most of the family arrived. Leading the way was my grandmother, Mom's 92-year-old mom, all of her children, grandchildren, siblings, nieces and nephews, along with my mother and father in-law, Mom and Pop Cornish, Moms' best friend, Miss Louisa, and my sister friend, Janet, to round out the list of honored guests. Many of us hadn't seen each other in a few years, so it was difficult to stop hugging and loving on each other long enough to take the photo. Getting everyone to stop and pose was like herding cats. That day, our family earned the dubious honor of being the worst family group ever photographed by that company. We know this because they told us so just before we placed our photo order. Despite the insult, we have an amazing family photo to cherish for a lifetime.

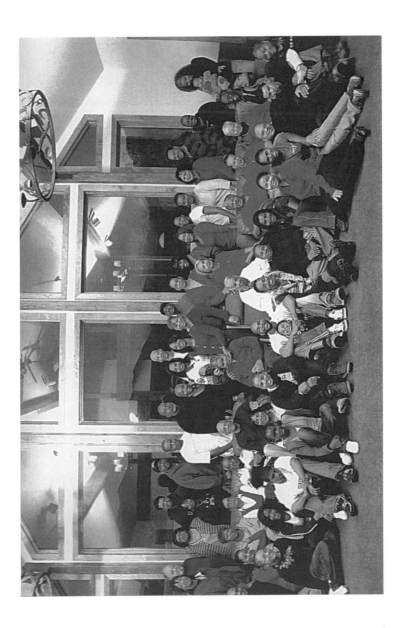

In true Colorado style, all weekend long we experienced brilliant sunshine, intermittent sleet and rain. The icing on the cake arrived in the form of snow. It would be a first experience for nearly half of our family. The wonder and beauty of the snow was capped off with the children, led by my fearless husband, spearheading a precision snowball fight with any unsuspecting relative who dared to venture outside.

In order to limit time spent in the kitchen, our dear friend from New Orleans, Chef Lisa of *Gourmet Away*, was hired to prepare family favorites, including jambalaya, red beans and rice, smothered chicken and gravy, stuffed peppers and crawfish etouffee. Did I mention the greens, candied yams, potato salad and baked macaroni and cheese? Each meal was topped with one of mom's favorite desserts, German chocolate cake, praline candy, Aunt Jannie's yam nut square, and bread pudding with the essential bourbon sauce.

Friday night was Mardi Gras themed, complete with purple, green and gold decorations, beads and carnival masks. We held a great big party filled with Mom's favorite music and lots of dancing. We each showed off our best dance moves and did our version of Mom's favorite steps. Mom had always been a finger snapper and a slow, smooth mover and groover. The laughter was loud and the joy was simply indescribable, erasing any thoughts of illness.

Saturday night was our chance to celebrate Mom exclusively and let her know how much we loved her. My mother always used to say, "Give me my flowers now while I'm here to enjoy them. Don't wait until I'm lying up there too proud to speak." We delivered the flowers while she could still enjoy them. We started out with a video of photos depicting her life. The entire evening was filled with great stories about Mom, some I had never heard. Over and over they demonstrated how generous, kind and selfless my Mother had been her entire life. We each got to share how much Mom meant to us and show her just how loved she was. This time, there was just as much laughter, but there were also plenty of tears.

On Sunday morning, we held our own church service. It was like an old time revival, full of wonderful singing and soul stirring testimonials. My uncles "T" and "Ike" did not disappoint as they sang Mom's favorites including, "It is Well with My Soul," "Another Day's Journey," and "Oh Happy Day." Cousins Vern and Tira provided their rendition of "Amazing Grace" while my sister Metrice and cousin Dominique gave us their rousing A&B selections. Joyful singing was followed by prayers of heartfelt thanksgiving as all of our family members and friends had survived hurricane Katrina. Indeed many of us had overcome extraordinary difficulties with the grace of Spirit. We each knew we were blessed beyond measure and expressed thanks and gratitude for all the obstacles we had overcome, especially for Mom. Sunday afternoon arrived too quickly and it was time for some of our family to head back home. Gratitude, a crucial ingredient for step three, **process**, shone down on all of us like sunshine, nurturing the resilience we would need for the rest of our journey.

The entire weekend had been the perfect "mountain top" experience and a wonderful celebration of my mother's life. How very grateful we were that Mom was able to experience and enjoy this occasion as we reflected on and celebrated the essence of who she was to all of us. Our trip to Estes Park, Colorado will go down in history as one of the best times we ever had together as a family.

After the celebration, we returned home and Mom was prescribed the hormonal drug Arimidex in hopes of shrinking the large, aggressive tumor. Arimidex did not work. When we knew it was time and nothing else could be done, we started hospice.

For weeks my mother had been asking to go home. Repeatedly, I told her she was home. The truth was, for nearly four years she lived with me and my husband in Denver, but Denver wasn't her home. Sacramento was her home, and it took me weeks to get it through my thick skull. When I finally got it, we made fast arrangements to take her back to California.

The warmth of the sun, familiar faces, family and friends would be just what Mom needed. Despite her prognosis, we were optimistic that a few months at home would be amazing. My brother Derrell and his wife Tina made their warm and homey cottage Mom's home. Her room was filled with photos and the eclectic collection of elephants she cherished. The room had a safari theme and the beautiful bay window let in just enough sunlight to glimpse the trees swaying in the wind.

When Mom and I arrived in Sacramento, hospice had already delivered the hospital bed and would come the next morning to meet with us. The nurse said Mom's vitals were good, and they would insure she would have no unnecessary pain. The first few days, Mom was unusually cranky and nothing we did seemed to satisfy her, despite having her beloved minister and church members visit and most of her kids and grandkids around. By midweek, she asked for her mother, the 92-year-old, feisty and sometimes cantankerous matriarch of the family. Before I could call my grandmother, she was calling to inform us she would arrive in 48 hours and we had better not be late picking her up from the airport.

Two days later, my sister Metrice came over early and dolled Mom up. Mom was glowing and beautiful. She had on her favorite soft peach gown. Her preferred lipstick, Rum Raisin, had been applied to her lips and a dusting of blush enhanced the natural glow she somehow still managed to possess. Her curly, salt and pepper hair framed her face like a halo.

When my grandmother arrived, Mom, with loving enthusiasm, said, "Hi Momma!" and gave her the most radiant of smiles. We were all taken aback as she hadn't smiled like that for any of us in days. Those would be my mother's last words. She slipped into a coma and took her final breath 72 hours later.

My brothers and I had made a pact a few years earlier. I would take care of Mom, but final arrangements would be their responsibility. They took care of the business, but as the oldest daughter, I had veto power and they ran everything past me. Mom's wake and funeral services were a Celebration of Life befitting the extraordinary woman she was, complete with a proclamation from the City of Sacramento and the State Legislature of California honoring her life.

Mom never liked to talk much about her final arrangements, but she let me know she preferred a crypt over a graveside burial. My brothers saw to it all of her wishes were met. There was one thing, however, they didn't tell me. When we arrived at the cemetery, to my great surprise, we were met by a brass band playing "Just a Closer Walk with Thee."

Following interment, the band played the traditional New Orleans second line music, "When the Saints Go Marching In." As is the custom for some New Orleanians, we danced and celebrated, knowing that my mother was now at peace.

Grief Was Impossible to Outrun

The following weeks and months were a blur. I had spent twelve years of my life as a caregiver and the last four years as a 24/7 caregiver and didn't know what to do with myself. The relief I thought I would experience simply wasn't there. All of the things I thought I had missed out on and had waited anxiously to be able to reclaim were no longer appealing. Grief was a constant companion, a rude interrupter and something I had no use for. I wanted to get this grieving thing over with quickly. Home, without my Mom, no longer felt like home. It would be unbearable when my husband left for work and was gone for his 24 hour shifts. The void was so palpable.

I traveled and ran as hard and fast as I could, but I couldn't outrun the grief. It met me around every corner, in every city and on every highway I traveled. Whether visiting family in New Orleans, taking a girls' trip to Florida, attending a graduation at Princeton or birthday celebrations in California and Pennsylvania, nothing felt right.

One day I received a call from my friend, Dolores. Her dad had been on dialysis and was rushed to the hospital. She was scared and didn't know what to do or where to turn. Her trembling voice was all too familiar. I met Dolores at the hospital and things didn't look good for Mr. Ross. I had met him before, and he was a very strong and dignified elder with mocha brown skin smooth as a glass of brandy. But now Mr. Ross had pneumonia and had suffered a stroke. When he was able to communicate a few days later, he told his daughter he was tired and didn't want to continue dialysis. His doctors recommended hospice and we began searching for options. As I companioned Dolores and her husband Derrick through this process, there was an energy surging through me that I had never felt before. I felt a purpose and a calling.

It was only a few days later when Derrick asked me to help with funeral arrangements. I wasn't certain I could. It was too soon after my mom's passing and I just didn't feel ready for a task of that nature. As I was about to say no, Derrick said, "We've never been through this before and it's just us." I knew with great certainty my purpose was to assist them, so I did.

In my research, I discovered Costco's online service provided caskets at a substantially reduced cost. Derrick was a practical man and appreciated the information and proceeded to order the casket from Costco at a very substantial savings. This helped us to coordinate a more economical, yet very beautiful funeral service for Mr. Ross.

Afterwards, I continued moving forward despite my own grief, uncertain where I was heading. I supported Dolores as best I could as we both learned that grief would not be ignored nor could it be rushed. I stayed busy, volunteered for political campaigns, looking for distractions any and everywhere. I got counseling and enrolled in not one but eventually, two different grief courses at two different churches. I was seriously looking for a magic bullet which did not exist.

It seemed no one I knew could understand the magnitude of the grief I continued to experience. My husband understood to an extent, but at the time, he had never lost a parent. Only those who have had similar relationships and similar losses could even begin to relate. I had been a long term caregiver to my mom, my friend, my rock, and all of that was now gone. I found myself bemoaning what could have been and should have been. My mom had spent the entire last decade of her life battling one series of illnesses after another, involving one obstacle after another. We missed out on so much of life together. It just wasn't fair and I was mad as hell about it.

A Birthday and the Holidays

Before I knew it, it was October, Mom's birthday month. On her birthday my husband was on a 24 hour shift at the fire station. I spent the day going from one movie theatre to another trying not to think. I immersed myself in the darkness of the theatre and the plot of the movie. No one could hear or see me cry.

Just as I thought grief couldn't get any heavier, it showed me it could. I thought the grief of Mom's birthday was unbearable, and now the holidays, an added reminder, were quickly approaching.

My husband and I decided to spend Thanksgiving in Seattle with my oldest brother and his family. The presence of family was a big help; however, the first holiday season without Mom was simply bizarre. Not being able to call Mom or hear her voice on a holiday was something I was unprepared for.

My love for all things Christmas came from her. In my world, my mother *was* the holiday, and now Christmas was looming. For the first time ever in my life, the thought of not going on and simply giving up emerged. I couldn't believe I was actually thinking such thoughts, but there were moments of grief that left me a shell of the person I had always known. Unwittingly, I had come to know despair.

Grateful for the love of God and my purpose in life, eventually I resolved to take the holidays full on and embrace what we had always loved. For Mom, for all of us, I was determined to make the holidays meaningful.

The first order of business was decorating the Christmas tree. I had all of Mom's favorite ornaments which would be placed on the front of the tree. Mom and I had very similar tastes so our combined collection of crystal and glass ornaments easily complimented each other. The hearts, lockets, hummingbirds and diamond drops were among our favorites. After decorating with the precision and intensity of a certified tree decorator, I stepped back to admire the dazzling, nine-foot tree adorned with all of the beautiful crystal ornaments, red flowing velvet ribbons and hundreds of twinkling clear lights. I had dreaded decorating this tree because I knew it would be emotionally excruciating. Even though the tears flowed nonstop, it turned out to be a cathartic experience. My mother would have loved that tree and I could hear her excitement and joy as I took in the scent of Douglas pine and the glow of white lights in the darkened room.

I placed the angel ornaments that had meant so much to Mom on a memorial wreath. As I hung the wreath on the door of her bedroom, the blue spruce prickling my fingers, an unexpected sense of solace laid itself over me like a warm blanket.

Louisiana Seafood Gumbo

Next was preparation of the gumbo. I wasn't ready to host Christmas dinner, but I would have my Boulder Briar Patch Book Club members over and I would cook Mom's specialty, Louisiana Seafood Gumbo. We're from New Orleans and she made gumbo like you would not believe. Her gumbo was the best I had ever tasted, and I vowed Christmas, 2008, I would master it.

Some say the tradition of Louisiana gumbo goes back to the early 18th century and is based on traditional West African native dishes. It is the most extolled and celebrated of all Louisiana dishes and is the hallmark of most special occasions in the region. People travel from around the world to New Orleans to experience this culinary extravaganza.

The most renowned gumbo is Louisiana Seafood Gumbo, which often includes shrimp, crabs and sometimes oysters. Vegetables include green peppers, onions, garlic, bell pepper and a small hint of tomato. Many add ham or tasso (spicy cured pork), hot sausage, chicken, andouille (Cajun spicy pork sausage seasoned with garlic) and smoked sausage. The secret to a great gumbo is the seafood stock and the base, or the roux, which is added at the beginning of the process. Additional thickening ingredients are included at the very end: filé (pronounced fee-lay), a powder made from dried and ground sassafras leaves, and/or okra, which can be floured and baked first so it thickens the gumbo. There are numerous variations to this beloved staple, but ultimately, they all aim to do the same thing—create a rich, intoxicating comfort food for the soul. Gumbo is the comfort food to end all comfort foods. It heals, it restores and it redeems.

The preparer of the gumbo ought to be as seasoned as it is, and should have some life experiences under his or her belt. The most revered gumbo is prepared in community and seasoned with the secret sauce, L-O-V-E. No matter the recipe, the sheer magic of gumbo is no two pots ever taste exactly the same.

Although I was well-seasoned with years of caregiving and months of grief, and although I had made many pots of gumbo in community, I had never before attempted making Mom's gumbo without her presence. Whether in person or over the phone, she always provided direction, fussed at the healthy alternatives I wanted to use, and often complained if I didn't do things exactly as she said to do them. I was immobilized over the thought of taking on this task without her.

In her absence, I contacted my grandmother and my mom's sisters for tips. Their input was essential. I needed to have Mom's spirit in the room this holiday season. I was coming to the realization that I was no longer sure who I was without her. Funny thing was my aunts all had their own variations of the perfect pot of gumbo. Somehow, I would figure it out. I was convinced that making gumbo and making it perfectly would be the only way I'd get through the holidays. I moved forward with the confidence of a highly insecure person.

I did the necessary shopping. I already had the seafood in the freezer from my recent trip to New Orleans. At the appointed hour, I chopped, I diced, I peeled and deveined the shrimp, and I sobbed and mourned. By the time everything was prepared, the big pot had come to a rolling boil with all of the seasonings. I began the task of preparing the roux. Mom would always say, "It should be dark caramel, but never, ever let it stick or burn." I was flooded with wonderful memories as I worked and tried in vain to hold back the tears.

As I diced and chopped and cut and stirred, my mind drifted to a memory that my heart needed in that solitary moment. A couple of months following Mom's stroke, four years before she died, my sister Metrice, sister-in love Tina and best friend El all gathered together in the kitchen to make a pot of gumbo. Mom was in her wheelchair giving orders about what we needed to do, how to do it and when to do it. It was a lot of hands and a whole lot of secret sauce that went into making that special pot of gumbo, which was exceptional, as, of course, were all those that followed.

This Christmas however, I was alone and on my own. The roux was done, the pot was boiling and all the necessary base ingredients had been added. I simply needed to wait and see. I sampled a taste to see if I was on the right track. Oh my gosh, it was a mess! The gumbo stock tasted horrible! It was bland and actually had a bitter tinge to it. I had no idea what I had done wrong. I adjusted the pot to a low fire, left the kitchen, went to my bedroom and collapsed on the bed. I was alone, distraught and in physical and emotional pain over the failure. Somehow, I had managed to ruin Mom's cherished gumbo!

I set the alarm so I could check the pot in another hour and fell into a deep slumber. I didn't even hear the alarm go off. I awoke, in a complete panic, sniffing the air for the horrific scent of gumbo gone wrong.

As I came to my senses, I realized what I smelled wasn't a burnt pot of gumbo at all. No, the aroma was magnificent. It was the scent of all things right in this world, sunshine, blue skies and the kiss of a light sea breeze on my cheeks. It was the indescribable, incomparable smell of a hearty, delicious pot of seafood gumbo. While I slept, the seasonings had blended over the low heat and created a beautiful harmony of aromatic flavors and richness. Those in the know, *know* that you can tell how good a pot of gumbo really is based on how it smells.

The smell wafting throughout the house wasn't just good—it was divine. I was elated! Surely Mom had come to visit and blessed that pot. When I tasted the gumbo, I was overjoyed. I was literally tasting my mother's recipe! As I stirred the pot, tears streamed down my face and into the gumbo. These were not tears of sadness but of pure, unadulterated joy. I did my Happy Dance, y'all!

At that exact moment the voice I had heard a year earlier spoke again. It reminded me of *The Assignment*. The assignment I had received and had somehow forgotten about or ignored—to help other family caregivers in their quest to care for their loved ones in the home. It was the assignment I was certain of when my friends, Dolores and Derrick, asked for my help, the mission to be a sounding board and a support system for caregivers. This assignment was now so clear, to launch the business which would serve as a tribute to my mother, The Caregiver's Guardian, LLC.

**Weeping may endure for a night,
But joy will come in the morning.
Psalm 30:5**

I heard this scripture over and over again after my mother passed. I kept waiting for the morning to come. I wanted it to come much sooner than it did and when it finally arrived, I didn't want it to leave ever again. It did leave and to this date, in varying degrees, grief continues. After eight years, I suspect I will grieve the loss of my mother until my final breath. I am coming to terms with that, and I now give myself permission to feel what and how I feel. I now know the depth of my grief is correlated to the depth of my love and the unique relationship I was fortunate to have. It doesn't matter what anyone else thinks. This is my process, my journey, and is exclusively mine to bear. I used to be so ashamed of the tears. I have now learned to embrace them.

recipe card

Tears—2 Quarts

1. Allow tears to flow liberally and freely. It's OK!
2. It's a fact. Life is not fair.
3. For caregivers, grieving is part of the process which can begin at the moment of diagnosis or as soon as your loved one begins to decline. This is known as anticipatory grief.
4. Give yourself permission to grieve. Grieving time is unique to each individual and must be adjusted accordingly.
5. You cannot fast cook grief. It takes its own sweet time and may never, ever be done.
6. Identify that special ingredient, that special thing your loved one cherishes or covets.
7. If it brings them comfort, learn how to do it. It will comfort them and later it will comfort you.
8. God, Spirit, The Divine has answers for you. Ask, listen and answers will be revealed to you.

chapter two

Attitude Is Everything

It's not what happens to us in life that matters. It's how we react to what happens that determines success or failure.

When I began caring for my mother, I was fortunate to have a loving and supportive husband who was willing to help me do any and everything. My husband, Kevin, is a 6'4" tall drink of water, a basketball player in his college days. He is a firefighter and the epitome of cool. Nothing flusters him (well almost nothing). Yet even with his support, there were many days, especially the ones when he was working his 24 hour shifts, that were especially hard. This was due in part to my mom becoming partial to having him as her caregiver and being very difficult with me, loving daughter or not, when he wasn't around.

On those days, the thing that would get me through the hardest times was remembering that around the corner lived Miss Yvonne. She had the most positive attitude towards caregiving I have ever seen, and she embodied the powerful force of her love in a tiny, 4'6" frame. I had met Miss Yvonne a few years earlier, when I first moved Mom to Denver. We were on a walk in our quaint Orthodox Jewish neighborhood and I was pushing Mom in her wheelchair. Miss Yvonne stopped to introduce herself. Petite and energetic, her salt and pepper hair perfectly styled, she wore finely tailored clothes over her small frame, set off with a brightly patterned scarf. Her warm, bronze face was punctuated with two deep dimples which grew deeper every time she smiled, and that was most of the time. She introduced herself and shared that she too was a caregiver.

I would later learn she was taking care of her mother who had dementia and her brother who had multiple sclerosis. She did it every single day, with a smile on her face and nary a complaint. Miss Yvonne was a solo caregiver and had been doing this for more than ten years. She had clearly achieved mastery of step three, the **process**, and all it entailed.

I could not figure out how this little lady could take care of those two people and maintain not only her sanity but her love of life as well. As I got to know her, I saw that in her seventies she had the muscled arms of a body builder. She was a stylish dresser with classic taste and touches of flare. But aside from being with-it and smart, the reason Miss Yvonne did so well in her caregiving role was that she was *connected*. Miss Yvonne introduced me to my first valuable resource, the African American Caregiver's Support Group. There I would learn about many other resources, have a place to discuss my concerns and get to know people who really cared about each other and listened to one another.

The Importance of a Support Group

My first visit to the support group left me uncertain. My initial impression was most of the members were my mom's age and older. There didn't seem to be anyone there who was my age and who could identify with what I was going through. I had a new husband, a new job, was living in a new city with few friends and had to care for my mom. Our lives revolved around caregiving.

The group's facilitator was Nedra Sanders, a handsome woman, tall in stature and large in her grace and elegance. She would eventually become a mentor and a friend. I was immediately impressed with her depth of knowledge and the genuine warmth and compassion she showed for all of the caregivers she interacted with. In spite of that, the group initially did not resonate with me because of the age differences. To my regret, it would be some time before I overcame my concerns and returned. I felt like a "lone ranger" who had been drafted for an assignment I didn't remember signing up for. I resisted the obvious community right in front of me, even though I was clueless and on a steep learning curve regarding caregiving. I still swirled around in the whirlpool of **helplessness**, and hadn't yet moved toward **recognition** of what the caregiver's task entailed. Nor had I grasped the team approach which characterizes step three, the **process** of conscious caregiving.

Miss Yvonne was one of those people who always chose to find the positive in every situation. From her perspective, although her mother had dementia, her mom still managed to be joyous and peaceful. Miss Yvonne saw to it the long standing traditions her family held were maintained but modified based on the reality of their circumstances. Participating in civic and community events was still important and they would attend, they just wouldn't stay very long.

For months, I didn't understand how Miss Yvonne got her brother in and out of his wheelchair. He was so big and she was so little. One day, she revealed a male caregiver would come in twice a day to prepare her brother for the day and get him ready for bed at night. What a relief, because until then, I really thought Miss Yvonne was lifting and transferring her brother. I was questioning my own dexterity and strength as I pondered how in the world she did that. Miss Yvonne clearly knew how to utilize resources available to her in the caregiving community.

What I learned from Miss Yvonne was invaluable: attitude really, truly is everything. During an evening visit at her home, we were enjoying a glass of her favorite wine. As I marveled at her strength and the joy she radiated, I was compelled to ask, "How do you do it?" She said, "Caring for a loved one is a decision you make. It's about perspective. Every day you wake up and remember that ultimately, it is your decision to do this. You knowingly, willingly, take on the responsibility." Her dimples deepened as she smiled at me, coaxing me toward recognition of my situation and acceptance of it. "Your loved one didn't ask to be in the position that they're in," she said. "I always think about how I would want to be treated if I were in their shoes."

Late that evening, as I lay in bed and reflected on those words, I imagined, with a mindset of that nature, I could become a much better caregiver to my mother. It was clear to me with the right attitude it is pretty easy to do anything. And when you do what you do consciously and out of love, then it is made so much easier.

Miss Yvonne also said she did not believe in having pity parties, not for herself and not for her loved ones. She never looked at her loved ones through the lens of their afflictions. It was really a self-serving attitude. If she didn't pity them, she most certainly could not pity herself.

Years later, I could look back and recognize something remarkable had transpired. Miss Yvonne had been guiding me on the caregiver's journey, moving me along from **helplessness** to **recognition** of what the task was, recognition of the fact I had already signed up for it, and recognition of what I needed to be and do to succeed in it.

Time for Yourself Is Non-Negotiable

Miss Yvonne's one and only brother was her best friend and she loved him fiercely. She felt it was her honor to care for her brother, Isaac. Though wheelchair bound, Isaac was a strong man, with a chiseled face and a great big heart. He was socially conscious, loved politics and was concerned about humanity as a whole.

Her mom, Miss Lilly, was and had always been someone special. Even with dementia, she always had an endearing smile on her face. Miss Lilly was a lady of style and charm. Petite and loving, she always had a kind word for everyone. She affectionately referred to me and many others as "Sugah."

Miss Yvonne exemplified how important it was to do the things you still loved to do while caregiving. She understood the need for respite care and creating time for herself. She regularly got together with her old friends, went out to lunch, saw Broadway plays, and took in her favorite musicians when they came to town. She loved shopping and dining out and did those things as often as she could. Miss Yvonne always knew how to have a good time, and being a caregiver wasn't going to change that. She even had a group of friends who loved taking annual cruises to the Caribbean with her. She grew up connected, and stayed connected, no matter what challenge life threw her way. For Miss Yvonne, caregiving wasn't a burden. It was an honor.

As for me, I was exhausted. The joy and grace I wanted and needed seemed to elude me. Miss Yvonne, however, manifested an unparalleled grace. She was who I wanted to be when I grew up. When this would happen, I couldn't say.

When my mother passed away, Miss Yvonne was right there to support and encourage me. How did she do it? How could she do it? Where was her reserve and how could she give so much when she was already giving so much? A year later, with her support and encouragement, I would launch The Caregiver's Guardian, LLC (TCG). Six months later, I was at the hospital with Miss Yvonne when her brother died. She was grieving his loss and was not prepared for his transition. Even after caring for him day in and day out for twelve years, she was not ready for him to be gone. There was no solace for Miss Yvonne. Her brother's funeral would be the first of many TCG would assist in coordinating.

I would visit Miss Yvonne and her mom regularly after her brother's death. Seven months later, I would call and learn Miss Lilly had passed unexpectedly. Again, I would help Miss Yvonne coordinate a funeral for a loved one.

I am humbled by role models with character such as Miss Yvonne's. I could not imagine handling the loss of two people, two people I loved and cared for and lost in such close proximity to each other. Miss Yvonne exemplifed grace under fire and did so with a regal dignity. She honors her loved ones' memories and knows she did everything she could for them while they were alive. With regard to their deaths, she said, "Yes, I miss them dearly, but there are no regrets." She had given her all in love and caring, and she was satisfied.

I learned so much from Miss Yvonne. She has become both a mentor and mother figure to me. She embodies the very essence of who I aspire to be with her loving spirit, calm nature and incredible sense of knowing. The lessons I've learned from her about positive attitude and love are lessons I share with all of my clients.

Though all these things are vital, they aren't all you need to succeed as a caregiver. Miss Yvonne also took care of the fiduciary and legal responsibilities for her mother and brother. She understood **recognition** of the task included responsibility for the administrative duties as well. The task of getting the paper work in order is a vital one for everyone, not just for caregivers. We should all insure that our affairs are in order.

My oldest client, Miss Mellie, lived out the winter of her life according to her own wishes because she placed her affairs in order long before she thought it was necessary. Miss Mellie was clear on her options and prepared for the "just in case."

recipe card

Attitude Is Everything— 1.5 Pounds

1. Check the temperature of your attitude.
2. When you think your situation is hard or unbearable, look around. There is always someone else whose challenges and circumstances are more difficult than yours.
3. Taking care of others is not a license to self-neglect. You must take care of yourself first.
4. Do not stop living your life because you are caring for someone. Create a way to do the things that are important to you.
5. Stir the pot and remove any remnants of self-pity or pity for your loved one. Pity will not serve you or them.
6. Keep your dreams alive. You're never, ever too old to fulfill them. Garnish your reality with a sprinkling of dreams that warm your heart and make you smile.

chapter three

Affairs in Order, Check

Are you taking care of business? In the event of an unexpected illness or untimely death, will your loved ones grieve over the chore you've left behind for them or will they grieve for you?

I was always taken by the story of the famous Delany Sisters who lived to be over 100 years old. They became famous when their oral history, *Having Our Say*, stayed on the New York Times bestseller list for nearly three years. They were civil rights pioneers and educators, and they took care of each other until Bessie died at 104. Sadie lived until she was 110 and wrote her third book at 107. I couldn't have imagined one day I'd get to know a set of twins who would enamor me in the same way.

I met Kellie and Mellie when they were 88 years young. The twins had each lost their husbands years earlier. Kellie was active in church and was the cutest, spunkiest little lady you'd ever want to meet. Despite her age, she was a fashionista, keen and sharp-witted. At 90 she still walked the runway of the annual church fashion show and loved turning heads. Kellie was vibrant, enthusiastic and, as she liked to say, "On fire for the Lord."

Mellie, her twin, was demure, quiet and had been recently diagnosed with Alzheimer's. She would often point to the one deep dimple on her left cheek and whisper, "This is the one thing that I have that Kellie doesn't have, but I'd give it to her if I could."

We met in an elevator at church on a Saturday afternoon. I knew instantly Kellie was a caregiver. Kellie had the look in her eyes all weary caregivers possess, and she was eager to talk to someone who understood her plight. Kellie had two adult children and Mellie had one daughter. Kellie explained that she needed someone to help her plan for the care of her sister on a day-to-day basis. Intuitively, Kellie saw that I could help her move out of the weariness of unconscious caregiving and into empowerment through **recognition** of the caregiver's task.

Kellie talked about how close she and her twin sister had always been. She relayed the story of how, years earlier, she had gone to Pittsburg to visit Mellie, whom she had not seen in quite a while. When Kellie arrived at her sister's home, she was surprised to see her sister had the exact same living room set and bedroom set she had at home. Though hundreds of miles apart, they still had the same taste and preferences.

After consulting with Kellie's son, we put a plan in place that allowed Kellie to hire a caregiver who would come in a couple of times a week. We later added an Adult Day Program twice a week so Mellie would have a place to go for her own social outlet. As predicted, at first, Mellie resisted, but eventually she got used to the idea of getting out of the house and having activities of her own, an important part of her long-term care therapy. Mellie looked forward to the attention she received at the Adult Day Program and grew quite fond of one volunteer in particular. Miss Pauline took a special interest in Mellie and would paint her fingernails with fun colors and tell her tall tales and engaging stories.

I also introduced Kellie to the Caregiver's Support Group I attended. By this time, I was sold on the value and importance of a support group for every caregiver. This provided an outlet where Kellie could learn from other caregivers as well as learn about additional resources available to her. Our next stop was the local chapter of the Alzheimer's Association. We needed to educate Kellie on this disease and provide tools to assist her as things became more challenging. The Alzheimer's Association is a necessary and valuable resource for anyone dealing with any form of dementia. The local chapter of the Association has a 24-hour help line available that Kellie was able to utilize.

Kellie was keen on taking care of Mellie by herself and only asked for help whenever she really needed it. They had a sister in Nevada who would come out periodically to help, and once or twice a year they would go out to visit her. This allowed Kellie a much needed respite, time to travel and to do the things she wanted to do.

During one of their visits to Nevada, Mellie's daughter said she wanted to take her mom to church. Unfortunately, Mellie's daughter had a history of mental illness and there had always been concern about her motives regarding her mother. On this particular Sunday however, she was allowed to take Mellie to church. The time came for their return and there was no sign of them. The daughter did not respond to phone calls and she would not respond when family members appeared at her home.

She had barricaded herself and her mom inside the house, and it became necessary to contact the authorities. Mellie's nephew, Dave, took on the role of mediator, attempting to reason with Mellie's daughter. The police would not get involved because there was no legal paperwork. Resuming contact after 48 hours, the daughter informed family members she would be taking care of her mom. The family's more immediate concern was the daughter had none of her mom's medications, clothing or medical supplies. Meanwhile, Kellie, who had been enjoying several days of respite back in Denver, called me frantically, asking for help. We sought legal counsel and learned we would have to petition the Denver Probate Court for emergency guardianship. In this case, an attorney would be required. We hired an excellent lawyer who quickly got the wheels in motion. After three days of barricading herself and her mother, Mellie, inside the home, the daughter responded to her cousin Dave's gentle pleading and rational arguments, and released Mellie. That very day, Mellie and Dave were on a plane back to Denver.

At the age of 89, Kellie petitioned for guardianship and conservatorship for her sister, Mellie. A court visitor came to the home to conduct an assessment and determine whether Kellie had the capacity to care for her twin sister. The court visitor left duly impressed.

Kellie also had to pass a background check and provide a credit report. Mellie's physician provided the necessary documentation and medical records to verify her diminished capacity. The attorney and I were astonished as Kellie explained the finances—bank accounts, expenses, savings and retirement accounts—off the top of her head.

Kellie was astute and very clear about the court proceedings and what would transpire. The day prior to the court hearing, we learned Mellie's daughter was counter-petitioning for guardianship of her mother.

The daughter arrived in court with her own attorney and asked the judge to allow testimony from her adult children via phone. The judge allowed the testimony, and it was no surprise that her children would argue their mom was in a better position to take care of their grandmother. When the judge asked the daughter why, for the past ten years, had she not been taking care of her mother, the daughter could not offer an answer.

The attorney called Kellie to the stand. She clearly and articulately explained to the judge it had always been her sister's wish that she be cared for by her twin sister. This was not only a verbal discussion between the two of them. Ten years earlier, Mellie had completed the Power of Attorney (POA) paperwork naming her sister as her POA. The document stated in case of incapacitation and the need for a guardian or conservator, she named her sister Kellie as the responsible party.

I was called to the stand as Kellie's only witness, testifying to my work as her Care Consultant. I explained how Kellie and I had met at church, how I assisted her with hiring an independent caregiver and identified the best adult day care facility for Mellie. I also discussed the resources Kellie was using including the Alzheimer's Association and the Caregiver Support Group. Kellie had made the transition to conscious caregiving in step three, **process,** by seeking help and implementing it. Not least of the benefits of this step was the judge's approval of her team approach.

The judge was fair and allowed both parties to ask questions and present their cases. Mellie's daughter asserted her Aunt Kellie was simply too old to take care of her mom and made other allegations that were unfounded. Because of what I had been told by family members, I was rather surprised at the clarity of the arguments waged by Mellie's daughter.

In the end, the judge said whether she had an opinion or not, it really didn't matter. The statutes in the law were clear. First of all, Kellie was clearly capable of caring for her sister. Furthermore, Mellie had taken care of her legal affairs prior to becoming incapacitated. The court had no choice but to follow Mellie's wishes. Even if the judge wanted to give guardianship to the daughter, she could not because Mellie's legal affairs were in order regarding her desires, and her sister was capable of caring for her.

The judge then ruled in favor of Kellie becoming Guardian and Conservator for her twin sister, Mellie. The judge said she hoped if she ever needed care at 89, there would be someone like Kellie to care for her. Eighteen months later, Mellie passed away peacefully in her sleep.

Kellie is still living alone, content in her Independent Senior Living Community. I visited Kellie on her 94th birthday. She said it was a blessing that she was able to honor her sister's wishes and care for her. When I asked Kellie if moving to an Assisted Living Facility was something she was ready to think about, she said, "No, I'm pretty happy living here alone. Whenever I get lonely, I just go out front and sit on the bench and talk to all the people passing by. I wouldn't change a thing about my life." She ended the visit by asking, "Do you think I'm way too old to get me a husband?" I left listening to the sounds of her joyous and hearty laughter.

Most of us are not fortunate to have the special bond shared by twins. Mellie and Kellie were able to complete each other's sentences, and even when they lived in different states, would buy the same furniture and art work without each other's knowledge.

In Mellie's case, she knew getting her affairs in order was a must. Even as she and her sister advanced in age, she was clear about whom she wanted to leave in charge of her care. Not only did she know this in her mind and her heart, but she cemented her wishes by drawing up the legal documents to support her demands. A Living Will, Durable Medical Power of Attorney, Five Wishes Documents and a Will were some of the legal documents Mellie executed.

Prudence and sheer practicality were exercised by these twin sisters. Are your affairs in order? To neglect this task can result in upheaval for the whole family, not just danger or discomfort for the dying or infirm person, as Miss Florence's story makes painfully clear.

recipe card

Affairs in Order, Check— 2 Pounds

1. Check to be sure you have all of the necessary ingredients for yourself as well as for your loved one.
2. Fold in Power of Attorney, Durable Power of Attorney, Living Will, Will, and perhaps a Trust for yourself and your loved one. Find out if your loved one has Long Term Care Insurance. Read the policy for gaps and conditions of use. Weigh carefully the benefits of accessing that policy and use it while you can.
3. Itemize, then combine all of these essentials in a place for safe keeping. Inform two people you can rely on where these items are located.
4. Is your loved one's condition such, and are family dynamics such, that you should look into a Guardianship or Conservator for your loved one?
5. Legal documents are easy to ignore, but they should be the first ingredients on your list. Take care of it now!

chapter four

Family,
The Ties That Bind

The family we're born into is the family we have chosen.
We don't remember choosing them, but we did. Our families
teach us lessons no other individual or group can.

Catherine was at her wit's end when I received her call. Her mother, Miss Florence, was still living in the family home with two of her adult children, Sarah and Sam, both of whom had drug addictions. The house was becoming a revolving door for all types of shady characters, and Catherine wanted her mom out of that house. There had never been a discussion about what would happen in the event of such out of control circumstances placing her mother in danger. Catherine found herself alone, as no other family members were willing to intervene or step in to support her mom.

Catherine had already contacted Adult Protective Services (APS), but they had offered her no real solutions. According to them, there was no immediate threat although her mother had been diagnosed with Alzheimer's a couple of years earlier. Catherine learned that APS cannot always intervene, especially if there seem to be willing family members who appear to be competent caregivers when an investigation is done. APS always takes a least restrictive intervention approach. Catherine had already reached out to the local chapter of the Alzheimer's Association and had taken a few classes in order to better understand the disease and its course. Catherine's approach to her mother's situation showed grit and style, just like her surprising clothing choices and fun, colorful shoes. She was not stopped by a negative response from APS, but moved directly out of **helplessness** toward **recognition** of her task by gathering information about Alzheimer's.

Concern was increasing for her mother's health and diet. Catherine would prepare food daily, but she saw signs which revealed people other than her mom were eating her food. In addition, the house was starting to deteriorate. A reverse mortgage had been taken out on the home several years earlier. In Catherine's mind, the time had come to release the burden of this house and everything associated with it.

Exasperated, Catherine had nowhere to turn and was extremely grateful when a complete stranger referred her to The Caregiver's Guardian, LLC. Catherine needed to find a long-term care facility that would accept her mom. The process was lengthy and involved. She was shocked to learn the average monthly cost of a nursing home in Colorado was $7,000.00. She would have to begin by applying for Medicaid. Many people believe that Medicare will pay for the cost of long term care, but this is not the case. Long term care costs are covered via out of pocket expenses (cash) or by long term care insurance policies, but the policy must be in place well before the need arises.

Medicaid is an entitlement program designed to assist individuals with low incomes and few assets with the cost of long term care in the home or in a care facility. Applicants must meet specific income guidelines and must also have two deficits in activities of daily living (ADL's).

Miss Florence, who had always been ladylike in appearance, looked as though she had just left the salon. Now she could no longer bathe or toilet herself, nor could she prepare her own meals. She also used a wheelchair most of the time. She more than met the physical criteria for the program.

Approval for Medicaid also required written verification from her doctor. In addition, full documentation of expenses, verification of income and six months of bank account statements were required. My job was to help Catherine pull all of this information together and audit the completed application before it was submitted to Medicaid. She came to my office looking confused and disheveled, her mixed patterns not the style statement she had made in the past. Catherine was clear about her concerns but had no way of addressing them. By the time she left, she was standing five feet seven inches tall, had a clear plan, and exuded confidence and the willingness to implement the plan.

Importance of Power of Attorney

While all of this was happening, Catherine realized although she had Power of Attorney for her mother, in order to take care of the sale of the home and any other assets, she would have to petition for guardianship and conservatorship. Her siblings, Sarah and Sam, were unhappy about Catherine moving their mom (and themselves) out of the house, and they were livid over the petition for guardianship. I assisted Catherine in completing and filing the court documents. Because no one was contesting in court, an attorney was not required. When Miss Florence's son, Sam, decided to contest after all, he did not file the necessary response in time to speak during the court hearing. Ultimately, the judge ruled in favor of Catherine serving as guardian and conservator for her mother.

The next hurdle was identifying the appropriate care facility. It boiled down to which facility was in closest proximity to Miss Florence's children. We found one in walking distance to Catherine's home. Getting Miss Florence to agree to go was another matter. Miss Florence was quite stubborn and adamant she was not leaving her home. She had no plans whatsoever to live anywhere other than the address she had known for thirty years. She may have been in a wheelchair a majority of the time, but she was strong and knew how to use her cane to her advantage.

Catherine considered her options for transitioning her mother from her home. The facility would send an ambulance for Miss Florence, but they informed us if she wasn't willing to go, she could not be forced. There were concerns that Miss Florence's adult children might put up a fight over their mother being taken from her home, so a representative from Adult Protective Services, along with a police officer, arrived at the appointed time. Miss Florence sat fiercely upright in her wheelchair, her nails, hair and skin perfectly groomed as though she were going to church.

Over the course of my work assisting Catherine, I had developed a good rapport with Miss Florence, so it was decided I would do the talking to convince her to leave her home. I explained she would be taken to the clinic for tests and would get to stay there for a while. Miss Florence reluctantly agreed to get on the gurney, smoothed her skirt down over her stockings, and took the ride in the ambulance with as much aplomb as she could manage. As for me, my subterfuge is professionally referred to as "therapeutic fibbing," often a necessary tactic when dealing with individuals with memory impairment.

The first day or two at the new residence were pretty good ones for Miss Florence as she began to adjust to her new environment. But after a couple of days, she became extremely agitated and demanded to go home. As her behavior escalated and she became more threatening, she was placed in a mental health facility for treatment. There she was evaluated and given medication to calm her. This experience was daunting, and Catherine agonized over the decision she had made to place her mom in a long term care facility.

A week later, however, Miss Florence arrived back at the nursing home having made some adjustments to her new medication regimen. What Catherine learned was that even though she had placed her mom in a facility, there were multiple variables in the adjustment process before things would run smoothly. Patience, vigilance, assertiveness and a proactive mindset would be necessary attributes that she would have to learn. Catherine realized the complexities and challenges of caregiving could arise no matter where the care was being provided.

Conflict Escalation

Catherine is the first to admit she was under a great deal of stress at this time. Sleep deprived, she was plagued with guilt about moving her mom into a nursing home and rendering a brother and sister essentially homeless. Things got even worse when she and another sister got into an actual fist fight at the nursing home. An argument escalated, accusations flew, and before Catherine knew it, she was in combat with her sister—two grown, intelligent women going at it in public. The fight resulted in an arrest and Catherine was mortified to learn that her sister, the accountant, took advantage of this opportunity to file charges. Catherine would later take a plea bargain and agree to enroll in anger management classes. Regrettably, it was the interventionist who now required an intervention.

This entire process proved to be an expensive and valuable lesson for Catherine. She learned the importance of self-care, self-control and how crucial it is never to give your control or power to anyone. To be successful at step three, the **process**, conscious caregivers must find a way to manage both the situation and their high levels of stress. As Catherine discovered, either you learn to manage the stress or it will manage you.

Over time, Miss Florence slowly got used to her new home at the long-term care facility. The unexpected death of her daughter, Sarah, was the catalyst for reconciliation among the siblings. Sarah died quickly from ovarian cancer. Her death was a shock to the entire family but did not spur greater involvement by Miss Florence's other children.

The family is one of society's most complex entities. Parents can raise children with similar values and because each person is an individual with the power of choice, they can all choose different paths. All families have some level of dysfunction. The key as a caregiver is to recognize what you have control over. In most instances, the only thing that you can control is your reaction to the circumstances and scenarios you find yourself involved in. In Catherine's case, she made a decision to defend her mother against two of her siblings. In the process of doing so, her own imperfections came to light, and she was ordered to get help for herself as well. The multi-layered nature of the interventions required in this family demonstrates that there is help available from outside the family and a safety net provided by society. Difficult situations like Catherine's can be remedied, but may not always completely heal.

Catherine came to understand that in order to insure her mother received quality care in the long-term care facility, she would need to demonstrate how she wanted her mother cared for. She was vigilant in visiting her mother on a regular basis but did so at various times of the day. This kept the staff on their toes as they never knew when she would show up. It also helped to insure her mother received the attention she needed.

Unlike the families with intense connections portrayed so far, Miss Sue was completely isolated. She reached out for social services all on her own, but it seemed there was no one listening, no one who cared enough to address a simple application error. Miss Sue knew she was experiencing an injustice and continued to ask for help. She eventually found The Caregivers Guardian, LLC, and the advocate who would help change her life for the better.

recipe card
Family, The Ties That Bind— 2 Bushels

1. There is no such thing as the perfect family, and you will never create or find a recipe for one.
2. God gave you the family you have for a reason. What lesson is your family teaching you?
3. What is your plan if you can no longer care for your loved one in the home?
4. If you care for a loved one in their home, is a reverse mortgage an option that you and your loved one should consider?
5. What does your self-care plan look like? Coat it daily with an activity that demonstrates your love for self.
6. Your responsibility to your loved one is to insure they receive the best care possible. There may come a time when the demands outweigh your ability to provide that care. Identify the best place for them to receive care.
7. When a long term care facility is necessary, it is important that you model how you want your loved one cared for. The more you visit, the more engaged you are with your loved one's care, the higher the level of care they will receive.

chapter five

Advocacy

*I will be your voice when you have no voice. I will ask
the tough questions. I will do the homework and
the research because if the shoe were on the other foot,
you would do it for me.*

Caregivers must become advocates for their charge. Family caregivers wear many hats, and one of the most important ones is advocacy.

When I met Miss Sue she was battling cancer. Miss Sue was small in stature and reminded me of "Ma" (Sophia Petrillo) from the Golden Girls, both sharp tongued and sharp witted. By the time I met her, however, she was weakened by cancer and depleted by her fight with Medicaid. She called me because she had applied for Medicaid and had been denied even after appealing the decision. During her appeal meeting, Miss Sue had to carry her own trash can with her because she was so sick due to her chemo treatments. Even in that state, the supervisor listening to her appeal showed no empathy, simply told her she was not eligible, offered no explanation as to why and dismissed her. It made my blood boil just to hear that someone so visibly ill could be treated so callously. I was eager to learn more about the circumstances leading to this conclusion as I was convinced there had to be more to the story.

At the time, I only knew the very basics about Medicaid, but I thought I knew enough to help Miss Sue. I agreed to assist without charge and we would both learn together. The first thing I needed to do was review her application and supporting documentation. Based on what she told me about her finances, a monthly income of $1,100 and no assets, it didn't seem reasonable that she would be denied. After auditing her application, I could find no reason to warrant her denial. However, I did see Miss Sue had checked the box for Medicaid but had not checked the box for Medicaid Long-Term Care. Surely this would not be the reason for the denial. Even if it were, certainly during the appeal process she would be told that she needed to check the correct box, wouldn't she?

We immediately began the process of re-applying. We applied for every single program and made sure that all boxes were checked with a big X for each program. I audited each line to insure accuracy. We triple checked that every document requested was supplied. We hand delivered all documents into the Medicaid office and received verification for each document submitted.

Finally Approved

It may have been because I made a point to speak very nicely to every case manager as well as to explain what Miss Sue had already gone through. Perhaps it may have been someone involved in the process recognized an egregious wrong had been done. In any case, Miss Sue's application was the fastest approval I've ever secured for a client. Within ten days, the assessment for Miss Sue's long-term care needs had been conducted and approved. Within three weeks, Miss Sue's application for Medicaid Long-Term Care had been approved, and she also received a subsidy for her Medicare Monthly Premium. The look on Miss Sue's face when we received the news was priceless. She exuded gratitude for the fast correction that occurred and insisted that she pay a small fee for the advocacy service I had provided.

Miss Sue is an example of a patient who had to take charge of her own caregiving. She moved from **helplessness** at her denial by Medicaid, to **recognition** that the task with the bureaucracy required help from a Care Consultant, to a **process** where her caregiver (her daughter) could receive compensation. Miss Sue's quality of life changed dramatically and immediately. She received the home health care services she needed as she continued her battle against cancer. Her daughter received a stipend for the care she was providing her mother. Bills that had been accumulating for surgery, hospital stays and doctor visits within the previous 90 days were all covered by Medicaid. Out-of-pocket expenses for expensive cancer drugs were all reduced to a two-dollar co-pay, and Medicare monthly premiums were now covered by the Medicare Savings Program.

Miss Sue was happy, grateful and felt incredibly blessed. She became teary eyed each time she saw me and expressed her thanks and appreciation over and over again. I was simply thrilled an apparent wrong had been righted. I kept in touch with Miss Sue and her daughter on a regular basis to ensure no hiccups developed. None did. Even though her daughter wasn't available, Miss Sue attended my first Christmas gathering for caregivers and was thrilled to be a part of it.

A Heartbreaking Outcome

Then came a change. A couple of months passed and I didn't hear from her. I tried phoning and the number was disconnected. I sent a card and a couple of weeks later the card was returned to sender. I went immediately to Miss Sue's apartment and found no one living there. I was baffled. Where could she have gone?

I would later reach out to the cousin who had referred her to TCG and learn Miss Sue had died two months earlier. I was in shock. The last time I saw Miss Sue, she was beating cancer—she was winning.

Helping clients was what I did, but losing clients was not something I was prepared for. This loss really hurt. I gave myself permission to feel those emotions and be okay with them. Now it gives me solace and comfort to know that the last 18 months of Miss Sue's life were made a lot easier because she received services she desperately needed and truly deserved.

Miss Sue's story will forever be a reminder to me that "No" does not and should not always mean "No." Whether the obstacles you face are personal or bureaucratic, asking for help when you're uncertain is often necessary. It may lead you to a different outcome and/or a more favorable conclusion. In the case of bureaucracies, systems may appear to be designed to eliminate individuals from the process; a 32-page application can surely be a deterrent. Questions may not be clear and the responses received may not be clearly defined or understood. In these instances, it is prudent to ask for assistance. If you don't get the help that you need, find an advocate, someone who knows the system and has some experience. Merely having another set of eyes review the paperwork can sometimes offset potential, life-impacting problems.

As I've gained more experience with Medicaid and Medicare, I'm happy to report that this was indeed an isolated incident and the case managers and supervisors I've gotten to know over the years are indeed committed to helping clients navigate the application and recertification processes.

Miss Sue was a lone ranger in her process and she touched my heart in a meaningful way. However, it was Will and Teepa who demonstrated that love and the support of family have no boundaries. They showed me that the power of a loving couple can transcend anything. The love they had for each other and the love they instilled in their children shone a bright light for all to see and experience.

recipe card

Advocacy—Two Quarts

1. Dealing with the bureaucracy (Medicare, Medicaid, Social Security, long-term care insurance companies) can be challenging. If you are not getting the results you need, first ask for help within the system. If that help isn't provided, seek help outside of the system.
2. Ask questions, and if you don't get an answer you like, ask someone else.
3. Medicare will not pay for long term care costs.
4. Medicaid receives federal funding and is a state-run entitlement program that pays for long-term care for low-income individuals. Find out if your loved one is eligible.
5. "No" may be the first answer you receive. Do not accept that answer if you believe it should be a "Yes." Appeal is often a necessary ingredient. It's your right. Take advantage of that right with Medicaid, Medicare, Social Security, insurance companies and hospitals.
6. As a caregiver, learn all you can about your loved one's illness. You are their advocate, their voice, their eyes and ears. Soak in this knowledge until it becomes second nature to you. Take notes, use a recorder, ask questions, and advocate on behalf of your loved one.

chapter six

Salt of the Earth

Be kind. Be decent. Treat others fairly. Put God first.
And always remember to look up to the sky and
give thanks every day.

I never fully understood the meaning of the term "salt of the earth" until I met Will and Teepa. They were two of the most honest, caring, hardworking, God fearing people I have ever known. They lived their lives by the Word of God and aspired to enact God's word without ceasing. They strived to be good and decent people and enhanced the lives of those they encountered.

When I received the call from their son, he told me I had been referred by someone at a church I had never heard of. When we met, he confided, "I don't know what I don't know." He said his parents needed a lot of attention. All of the children lived out of state and their parents were adamant about staying in their home. Basically, he said he needed someone to be him—his eyes and ears—when he wasn't there. I was immediately impressed that this long distance caregiver had already moved out of **helplessness** about his parents' condition and into **recognition** of the size of the task ahead. He was ready to implement a caregiving **process** by assembling a team to meet his parents' needs.

I assured him I would work hard to be the best possible care consultant, and that operating in excellence was my goal. We didn't know it then, but this was the beginning of a three-year relationship which remains one of the most meaningful experiences I have been blessed to share.

Twenty years earlier, in her sixties, Teepa suffered a massive heart attack at home. Will called 911 and performed CPR. The paramedics arrived and immediately went to work but could not revive Teepa. Will stepped in and continued CPR. He wasn't going to quit and he was not ready to let Teepa go. When they arrived at the hospital, Teepa was placed on life support. Family arrived and they all knew the inevitable, everyone but Will.

No matter what anyone said and in spite of the fact Teepa had a living will and had said she didn't want to be on life support, Will would not take Teepa off of the machines. His persistence and bullheadedness paid off. Prayer was his constant companion, and eventually, slowly, Teepa began to come around. At first, she was not at all herself and had to relearn everything. Patiently, Will helped her learn what she needed to know. He took care of her with everything he had. Teepa was the love of his life and he was willing to do whatever it took to care for her. Her recovery was a long and arduous process. Some would argue she never completely recovered.

Teepa reminded me of Eudora Welty when I first met her. She was a tall, willowy, pale woman with a crown of fluffy white hair and a gentle drawl. She was both elegant and shy, with an inborn graciousness developed over a lifetime of good manners. I asked her how she and Will met, and she replied, "The first time I saw him I was 17 years old and I said, 'He is my man, even if I never ever get him.'" She married her man in 1947.

It was 2010 when Will and Teepa became my clients. Will was in poor health and on dialysis. A home health agency had already been hired, and 24-hour care was being provided. Even with this assistance, there was no overall care management or coordination of services in place. There were a lot of medical appointments scheduled and quite a few things around the home needed attention. This would be my first case of this nature, and I knew I was up to the task.

Teepa was a true Southern belle. Her world revolved around Will and their family. I didn't know what she was like prior to her heart attack, but she was one of the most caring and thoughtful women I had ever met. Teepa had been a teacher and became a homemaker when her three children were born. Her life revolved around family, friends, and church. Teepa never complained. She baked great pies and loved collecting antiques and teapots. Taller than Will, Teepa was demure and ladylike. Her thin, white hair held a natural curl that framed her pale wrinkled face. At one time, she may have dressed to fit her role as handsome Will's wife, but by the time I knew her, it seemed that Will had been purchasing her clothes for her, and let's just say color coordination was not his strong suit.

Because of his long hours at the dialysis clinic, it was a week before I met Will. I was told he would be a hard one to win over. But inside a few days, both Will and Teepa had won my heart and in no time, as unlikely as it seemed, I had become a trusted and respected advocate.

Will had the voice of Zig Ziglar. I could close my eyes and listen to him speak and imagine I was having a conversation with one of my heroes. He had long translucent fingers with prominent veins and a full head of white hair. Pictures from the past showed him to be a strong, strapping man. By the time we met, he was wheelchair bound, unable to stand tall. Will weighed 110 pounds and didn't have much of an appetite.

What he did have was a heart the size of Texas and a mind sharp as a tack. He would have an occasional bout of confusion but would snap out of it with crystal lucidity. He never forgot the love he had for Teepa or his love of God and family. Principled and disciplined, Will adored routine. There was a time and place for everything. Material things never mattered much to Will. Practical to a fault, he insured he and Teepa had what they needed, but no more. The television was a floor model from the '70s, and their home was a two-story cottage with separate living and dining rooms. The action took place in the den. Will was very kind but could be very rigid and opinionated. Throughout the time we knew each other, politics remained the one topic off limits, and we agreed not to discuss it.

As Care Consultant, I attended Will's appointments and served as his advocate. I monitored his care and saw to it only the best caregivers were assigned to his case. I kept in regular touch with Will and Teepa's adult children, letting them know about any concerns I may have had.

We had great conversations when Will told me his life story, accomplishments, travels and tales about his work as a geologist. He also shared his regrets. Will taught me the importance of looking up every day and appreciating the cloud formations which Will described as God's incredible handiwork.

I made it a practice to inquire about end of life wishes and the necessary documents verifying those intentions. In Will's case, he had taken care of the legalities with a will but had not expressed his wishes to his children. I shared the Five Wishes document (also known as the Living Will with a Soul) with their children. Will would not discuss end of life matters with his children. I explained to them that this was rather common among their parents' generation. In time, Will shared those wishes with me and I recorded them. As for Teepa, he simply wanted for her to have whatever her wishes and desires might be.

For Will, Hospice Finally

We were all elated when we were told Will would no longer need dialysis because his kidney functions had resumed. This was great news but it would be short lived. Sadly, as I attended appointments with Will, it became clear he didn't have much time left. I arranged a conference call with his children and his doctor to talk about next steps. It was time to start hospice, but this was a conversation no one was willing to have. Will was dying and everyone seemed oblivious to that fact, especially Will. The family was united in step three, the **process** of caregiving for these two remarkable parents. Given their love and devotion to their parents, it was only natural for them to take some time to adjust to Will's prognosis and arrive at the caregiver's fourth step, **acceptance**.

Though worried about Will, my immediate concern was for Teepa. She seemed so fragile emotionally. I wasn't sure how she would process or handle her husband's impending death. I knew it was important for her children to be there to support her. What I will forever admire about Teepa and Will's adult children was their willingness to put the needs, wants and desires of their parents first. It was never about them; it was always about their parents and what was best for them.

After digesting the news of Will's prognosis, they all stepped up to the plate. Their daughter, the apple of Daddy's eye, along with her husband and their children, came out to spend a week and would come out again for Thanksgiving. Will's sons came out to visit with their families as well. The granddaughter who lived an hour away visited regularly and helped out as often as she could.

The hospice staff was incredible, providing support for the family, the caregivers and for Teepa. It wasn't clear to any of us if Teepa was processing what was happening. It did not appear she was. But Will, on the other hand, was in complete denial. He was not going to die anytime soon. He stayed strong for as long as he could and willed himself to endure the pain and hold on for Teepa.

Because he still had a small appetite, I asked if there was anything special he wanted to eat. Having lived for a while in Louisiana, he was especially partial to gumbo. Now a specialty of mine, I offered to prepare it for him. The next day, Will and Teepa got ready to feast on Louisiana Seafood Gumbo. Teepa was so excited she couldn't wait to dive into her bowl of gumbo and did just that. Will gave her a stern, chastising glance and said, "Teepa, we haven't said grace yet." We all laughed, blessed the meal and enjoyed the gumbo. In the early evening hour, I phoned their children to tell them it was time to come. I felt Will would hold on until their children arrived because he didn't want Teepa to go through his death alone. The following day, Will was in terrible pain and said he couldn't take it anymore. The caregiver asked if I would come to the house. I arrived and visited briefly with Will. Just prior to midnight, as his oldest son and only daughter walked through the front door, Will looked up to the sky for the final time.

It had been only six months since I had been introduced to Will and Teepa. It felt like a lifetime. I had learned and experienced so much with those two and had grown very fond of their family. In retrospect, I have only one regret. Will became a sad statistic I have now come to dread, a caregiver dying first.

I believe it was Will's devotion and the depth of his gratitude for Teepa's life which sustained him during his lengthy caregiving journey. Until the last year of his life, Will refused help and felt he could handle things on his own. This stance took both a physical and emotional toll on him. Unfortunately, it is a stance which is not uncommon among spouses who find themselves in the caregiving role. Will's self-sacrifice and untimely death highlight the need for caregivers to do more than devotedly walk down the long tunnel of their caregiving journey. If they can move through the step of **recognition** of the size of the task and create a sustainable **process** with help, they can then move toward **acceptance** of the inevitable. Will was monumental in his stubbornness and his devotion. The high cost was obvious to everyone in the caregiving circle.

Accepting help sometimes seems inappropriate to the caregiver because they believe, "I should be able to take care of my spouse by myself." But there is nothing in the marriage vows that says, "In sickness and in health, without any help." It is important for caregivers to recognize that, even as a spouse, when the demands of caregiving become too big, it is alright to ask for and accept help. This may be beneficial in reducing rates of sickness and death among caregivers.

A 1999 study in the *Journal of the American Medical Association* by University of Pittsburg psychologists Schultz and Beach posited that stressed older adults caring for spouses with dementia had a 63% higher mortality rate than non-caregiving peers.

In contrast, a 2013 study in the *American Journal of Epidemiology* found that over 3500 stroke caregivers had no increased rates of death due to their responsiblities. That's good news. They actually found that caregivers had an 18% reduced rate of death compared with non-caregivers. This study suggests that caregiving can give a spouse purpose and prolong their life. For the caregiver, a balance between love and duty must be maintained as circumstances change.

In my experience, I've seen the former more often than not. A number of factors, including socio-economic status, spiritual support, familial support, health status, self care practices and hiring of professional caregivers have been the deciding factors as to which way the pendulum may swing for the primary caregiver.

It was nearly impossible for Teepa to grasp that Will had died, and daily she would ask, "Where is Will?" She managed to cope on some days and fall into despair on others. Yet she learned that no matter how bitter the cup served, life eventually offers up a sweet dish of surprises.

recipe card

Salt of the Earth—2 Cups

1. Salt is an essential ingredient that is best used in moderation.
2. Your parents worked hard for the money they've earned. Should their money be used for their care or preserved for your inheritance?
3. Your parents have always served as "your parents." It can be very difficult for them to relinquish control to you or anyone else, but especially to their adult children. Often times their relationship with you is the only thing they can control, so they give it all they've got.
4. Most people want to stay in their home as long as possible. It takes proper planning, substantial savings and adult children or a designated party committed to carrying out the wishes of the elderly for this to be achieved.
5. Talk to your care recipient about their final wishes. If they won't talk to you, find someone they will talk to.
6. Long-term care is expensive. Plan now for your own long-term care needs.

⚜

chapter seven

Surprises and Miracles

There is nothing like a touch of spontaneity or just a
sweet little surprise to lift your spirits.

Learning to live life without Will was really tough for
Teepa. Because of her dementia, she would often forget
Will had died and would ask for him constantly. This was
emotionally hard for her children and her caregivers as well.
It was especially hard for Teepa as she would revisit news of
Will's death as though it were the first time she was hearing
about it. Initially, the caregivers and I would respond honestly
and confirm Will had died, resulting in emotional agony for
Teepa. Eventually, we would deflect the question by having
Teepa talk about Will. We would ask questions about how
they met, the places they lived and traveled to and have her
tell stories which seemed to diffuse the shock of his death.

Despite this major loss, Teepa was adamant she wanted
to continue living in her home. Her children were not sure
if that was best. We consulted with a psychiatrist who saw
Teepa on a monthly basis. Teepa was sure of two things: she
missed Will desperately and wanted to be with him, and she
did not want to leave their home.

Teepa continued receiving 24/7 care in her home. That
care cost more than $14,000 per month. In an effort to

streamline costs, we would eventually eliminate the agency and hire three exceptional, independent caregivers. It would take a while to put all of the components in place to make this happen, but once it was done, everyone was pleased with the quality of care Teepa was receiving.

Teepa's children took turns visiting which made her very happy. She was equally unhappy when it was time for them to leave. We tried to get Teepa involved in an Adult Day Program. She attended a few sessions, but she simply wasn't interested. The caregivers took her out routinely to shop, to lunch and tried to find things to engage her in the home. Reading the Bible, solving seek and find word puzzles, and listening to music were things that gave Teepa solace.

She no longer wanted to do any of the things that she and Will had done together and was losing interest in going to Bible study, women's group and other things she previously enjoyed. Teepa had one friend, Shirley, who would visit her routinely. We were all concerned, but Teepa was grieving and there just didn't seem to be much anyone could do to help her. We sought professional help through a geriatric mental health program in the community. The psychiatrist was effective in maintaining medications and Teepa seemed to enjoy talking to her. Those visits were beneficial for Teepa as well as for her support team and family who would attend the appointments whenever they were in town.

What Teepa did seem to enjoy was staying home and savoring the relationships she had developed with each of her caregivers. First, there was Angela, a veteran caregiver. She was brilliant, well rounded on a number of subjects, funny, outgoing and a hoot with Teepa. She always found ways to make Teepa laugh and usually managed to have an interesting tale or two to tell. Angela did impressions of family members and caregivers. Even I wasn't spared as a target. She would have us in stitches as she nailed people's mannerisms and expressions.

Jewel, a nursing student and immigrant from Somalia, was completely invested in Teepa's welfare and devoted to her. Tiny in size and height, she had the youthful look of a teenager. Jewel was very quiet but had a beautiful heart connection with Teepa. They didn't talk a lot, but they seemed to understand each other at a deep level. Jewel was a soothing, calming force for Teepa.

Last but not least, was May. May had had a very special connection with Will, so she felt especially connected to Teepa. Will was May's hero, and she was determined to fulfill his wish to care for his beloved Teepa. May's heart ached as Teepa grappled with the loss of her beloved Will.

May's Pregnancy

May was six months pregnant and had been reluctant to share the news of her pregnancy with anyone. She worried about not being available to care for Teepa and was concerned she might not have a job when she was ready to return from maternity leave. She was also concerned about being judged by everyone because she was an unwed mother. May had bonded in a special way with Teepa and she desperately wanted that relationship to continue.

I reassured May we had plenty of time to figure things out. On a routine evening check in, May phoned to report the evening had gone well. She told me Teepa had been agitated earlier but had calmed down, and they would be getting her ready for bed soon. May confided she wasn't feeling very well and was looking forward to winding down after Teepa went to bed.

My phone rang at 2 a.m. I was in a deep sleep and did not hear it. My husband nudged me and said, "Your phone is ringing." By the time I answered, I had missed the call. Caller ID showed the home health care office had phoned and I had also missed an earlier call from May. My first thought was, "Oh no, something's happened to Teepa."

The Miracle

When I phoned the agency, the on-call nurse yelled, "Nadine, it's about May. She's had the baby!"

"What do you mean, she's had the baby? The baby isn't due for another two and a half months."

"She went into labor at the house! She gave birth to the baby on the dining room floor at Teepa's house!"

Surely I was dreaming. "What?"

The nurse said, "I've been trying to get a replacement over to the house but I can't get anyone to answer their phone. The police are there with Teepa and will stay until someone arrives."

I told her not to worry. I could get over to the house in 30 minutes. I got dressed and raced to Teepa's home. When I arrived, sure enough the police were still there patiently waiting. They reported Teepa woke up briefly and went back to sleep. It did not seem to bother Teepa at all that there were policemen in her home. The officers reassured me both May and the baby appeared to be just fine. May delivered the baby by herself. By the time the paramedics and police arrived, the baby was in May's arms. Mother and baby had been taken by ambulance to the hospital.

Teepa was resting peacefully and I didn't disturb her. I looked around the house and sure enough, in the dining room was the evidence that a birth had taken place. The police didn't mind waiting for someone to arrive, but taking on chores wasn't in their job description. I did a quick clean up and decided professionals would have to take care of the carpet. By this time, it was about 4 a.m. and I couldn't wait for 5 a.m. to come because I had to tell someone what had happened. With the different time zones Teepa's children lived in, it would be easy to call them bright and early to tell them about the little miracle that had taken place in their parents' dining room.

My phone rang an hour later and it was May. She was calling to make sure someone was at the house taking care of her Teepa. She assured me she was fine and the baby, tiny as anything, was doing okay. She then gave me the blow-by-blow account of what had happened. I could not believe my ears as she shared how she went from taking a shower to feeling like she had an upset stomach. She went to the front door to get some fresh air and all of a sudden, her water broke and the next thing she knew the baby was coming. This all took place in a matter of a few minutes.

When I asked if she'd thought of a name yet, she said "I am not sure." I teased and said, "He should be called Speedy Gonzalez. One thing we knew for sure about this kid was he was fast." May had no idea who Speedy Gonzalez was.

By this time Angela arrived for her regular shift. Of course, she was surprised to see me. It was time to wake Teepa when I told her, "You're not going to believe what happened." As I relayed the events of the evening to both of them, Teepa was excited and very engaged. Her radiant smile and sense of humor returned and her response was, "All this excitement happened right in my dining room and I slept through the whole thing? I missed out on the miracle? That baby showed up without any help from me at all." She shook her white hair wonderingly as she focused for a moment on the miracle of life.

My next stop was the hospital. I needed to check on May and see this fast little baby with my own eyes. May was doing great. She still couldn't believe her baby was already here. I put on the protective outer garment and prepared to enter the Neonatal Intensive Care Unit. This precious baby was just a little larger than my hand and was connected to a feeding tube, oxygen and monitors. His vitals were strong. The nurses were predicting he would be off machines within seventy-two hours. He was a beautiful little thing and from all indications he was doing well and would be just fine.

Sometimes a surprise is a miracle in and of itself. This event provided a great distraction for Teepa at a time when a miracle was truly needed. I can still see the big smile on Teepa's face as she got to hold little Elijah for what would be the very first and the last time.

The gift of this event became a blessing for me, a surprise which shifted me toward **acceptance** of Teepa's grief and her inevitable passing. Life rarely happens according to the script we've written or anticipated. In our bleakest moments, the universe can offer us something completely unexpected. Something that takes us out of ourselves long enough to recognize no matter what's happening in our lives, there is always a larger plan at work.

We can also open up to the possibilities of experiencing the power of love from people who are in our lives for just a season. Professional caregivers are utterly amazing in what they can offer their patient. They offer a different type of love and a connection that can serve in ways which are sustaining and will bless the patient, the caregiver and the family.

As mere mortals, we control so little in our lives, but at times we behave as though we are completely in charge. Those of us who really understand this know that the power of prayer, like nothing else in our lives, can and will change things. Dahlia demonstrated the power of prayer by using it in every facet of her life, especially in caregiving.

recipe card

Surprises and Miracles—2 Pints

1. You can't always know for sure what the right thing or the best thing is for your loved one. They are entrusted into your care. Make an informed decision based on what you believe is in their best interest. Follow your gut instincts. Use your intuition and improvise when necessary.

2. Joy comes in the most unexpected packages and can arrive at any time. Toss in as much as your pot can hold and stir frequently.

3. A miracle is a mystery ingredient which shows up when one is receptive and open to the possibility. Embrace the miracle as it adds texture and enhances flavor.

4. Learn coping strategies that won't traumatize your loved one with dementia. Reliving an event over and over, such as a loved one's death, need not occur when the caregiving team comes up with creative solutions like diversions and stories.

5. Even the greatest chefs seek guidance from a master chef. If you're dealing with dementia of any kind, your local Alzheimer's Association is a most valuable resource. Use it.

chapter eight

Praying Power

Understanding the power of prayer is one of life's most rewarding gifts. Many know how to talk to God, but grace comes in knowing when and how to listen.

Janie could be called a prayer warrior. She fervently believes in the power of prayer and will pray at any time for anyone. Curvy and vibrant, she maintains a commanding presence. Janie had a dream. She wanted to care for the elderly in her home, and she already knew what her business would be called: The House of Grace. Her business would have to wait, but her house was already a home of grace as Janie and her mother, Dahlia, took care of the matriarch of the family, Dahlia's mother and Janie's grandmother, Sarah.

Sarah exuded confidence and a strong will. She had piercing dark eyes, baby smooth skin and a Hershey's chocolate complexion. She was no longer speaking, but her eyes told you exactly what she wanted and needed. Sarah had fallen and broken a hip. She survived the surgery just fine and was sent to a skilled care facility for rehabilitation. The problem was there just wasn't much rehabilitating going on. Like many skilled care facilities, it also was housed under the same roof as a long-term care facility. Perhaps for this reason, there appeared to be little incentive to rehabilitate Sarah. Despite the family's daily visits to care for Sarah themselves, get her up routinely and keep her going, there just wasn't much cooperation on the part of the staff at the facility.

The family contacted me after several weeks of trying to get rehabilitation services for Sarah. When the skilled care facility continued to ask them to sign papers, alarm bells went off. The facility had transferred Sarah, without the family's consent, from skilled care into nursing care. This happened despite the family repeatedly saying they wanted to bring Sarah home as soon as she was able to come home. The staff informed the family Sarah could be better cared for in the facility and could provide the family a much needed break.

At 86, Sarah was in good health and her dementia afforded her a very easy-going and pleasant disposition. In other words, Sarah was no trouble at all. She was an easy patient and the nursing home wanted to keep her there. Appalled by this realization, the family immediately took Sarah out of the facility and brought her home. This family had already moved through **recognition** of Sarah's condition and into a caregiving **process** with professional help. They realized the help offered was not nurturing for their beloved Sarah. They were right to question the authoritative guidance offered by the nursing home. At some level, they understood there was a conflict of interest motivating the professionals who were advising them Sarah needed to be in their care, not at home in the care of a loving daughter and granddaughter.

The Unexpected

Two weeks later, Dahlia opened a bill from the nursing home totaling $10,000 co-pay for two months of care. The nursing home demanded that Sarah's full Social Security income of

$700 a month be applied to offset the bill. At this rate, it would take years to pay off the debt as Sarah had other obligations including paying rent. Despite the fact that Sarah had never signed papers, nor had her daughter, Dahlia, authorized any services, the charges mounted with monthly interest fees. The nursing home wanted Dahlia to sign a promissory note, taking responsibility for her mother's bill.

When I met with Dahlia she was quite upset. The good news was that Dahlia had not signed any of the paperwork, and best of all, she had not signed the promissory note they were pressuring her to sign.

Dahlia and I had known each other for a while. I was relieved to see that her skin had returned to a healthy glow and she no longer wore the exhausted demeanor that settles from the routine of providing twenty-four-hour care. She had entered the **process** of caregiving, realizing that it was not a solo journey, and had solicited and accepted help from other family members.

The first thing we needed to do was to contact the local Ombudsman for the nursing home. That person's job is to mediate any disputes and address complaints that are filed by patients and their families. The next thing we did was to contact Medicaid to find out what recourse Dahlia and her mother had through them.

The Ombudsman scheduled a meeting at the nursing home. Prior to the meeting, Dahlia and I met. Dahlia was so nervous it was infectious; she made me nervous. Truth be told, I was feeling a bit of tension because this was the first billing dispute of this magnitude that I had handled.

I asked Dahlia if she wanted to pray before going into the meeting. Dahlia said she was so relieved I had offered to pray, she could have cried. The prayer had a wonderful, calming effect on both of us as we proceeded into the meeting.

The financial representatives were there along with the acting director of the care facility. We explained what had transpired and stated Sarah simply did not have the funds to pay the bill. The family believed Medicaid would fully cover the cost of her stay in the skilled care facility, because they had never been informed otherwise

During the time of her stay, Sarah still had her share of the financial obligation for the home she shared with her family. Had the family known Sarah was accruing a debt, they would not have had her stay in the facility. They had no knowledge that a bill was accruing because somewhere along the way, the necessary paperwork had never been provided to Dahlia, who had Power of Attorney.

Though everyone was cordial, we did not come to a consensus. We explained again Sarah's limited income would not allow her to cover the cost of such a large bill. Dahlia told them that it was impossible to "get blood from a turnip." At the very best, a payment plan of $50 a month could be offered out of Sarah's limited income. The offer was not accepted and we left the meeting with nothing resolved.

The nursing home continued to send a bill every month, and Dahlia continued to collect the bills and place them neatly in her special box and pray over them. The box was black, embossed with an antique gold weave. The interior had a soft, black velvet lining. Dahlia called the box her prayer box and inside the box, she placed all things that needed Spirit's care. Dahlia was familiar with **surrender** in all aspects of her life as she had long ago surrendered her life to God's care and love. She readily practiced surrender in the act of caregiving for her mother. For this, she was exceptional among the caregivers I have known.

Like clockwork every month, Dahlia received a past due statement demanding payment. On the sixth month, Dahlia received the monthly statement, but this time there was something different. The statement indicated there was a zero balance due. No explanation was ever provided by the nursing home or Medicaid and none was ever requested.

Janie and Dahlia believe fervently in the power of prayer. This ritual has sustained them in the most difficult times and has served them well as they continue to provide 24/7 care for Sarah. For reasons no one can explain, the dementia is especially kind to Sarah and she is in a constant state of ease and peace. Janie and Dahlia pray daily, and I can attest that their prayers have resulted in a loving, quiet and peaceful household that indeed feels like "The House of Grace." May I say also that the very action of prayer produces results.

This family exemplifies the epitome of living and walking in faith. They recognize God, their higher power, has the capacity to handle whatever they are willing to turn over. Not only does this change the outcome, it impacts their process. I have witnessed firsthand the release of earthly concerns to Spirit. This allows the elimination of undue stress and anxiety, regardless of the circumstances. Paradoxically **surrender** is empowering. It allows resilience to blossom like wildflowers in a field.

Prayer and meditation are some of the highest forms of self-care. Taking intentional and dedicated time for oneself, breathing deeply, enjoying walks in nature, soaking in a hot bath with candles, singing, listening to uplifting music, even dancing, are all ways to surrender, maintain self-care and thus provide better care to the loved one.

Janie, Dahlia and their family have created an effective and cooperative team to care for Sarah. They accept support and have come to recognize that great care is best provided by a collective body. In this instance four generations come together to support the matriarch of this exceptional family. More broadly, the concept of caring for each other is alive and well among them.

The power of acceptance is further demonstrated by my personal story about coming to terms with the necessity of a full team to assist in caring for my mom in the final stages of her life, and my surrender to her passing on to the next.

recipe card

Praying Power—Generous Dosage 2 to 3 Times Daily

1. If your loved one is in a skilled care or long-term care facility, identify who your Ombudsman is. If and when needed, add their assistance to your skillet. Their contact information will be posted on a bulletin board at the facility. If you have a problem at the facility that isn't resolved, contact the Ombudsman directly and immediately.

2. As a caregiver or Power of Attorney, you are not personally liable for bills or debt incurred by your loved one. You are only responsible for paying debts that have been incurred on your loved one's behalf from their own resources. Always sign any documents or statements on their behalf with your name and POA in parenthesis.

3. No matter what your religious preference or practice, creating a ritual of prayer and meditation is essential for your spiritual, mental and emotional wellbeing.

4. If you don't know Jesus, now may be a good time to find Him.

5. Prayer changes things. It creates inner peace and dissolves chaos. Whisk in frequently.

⚜

chapter nine

Teamwork, It Works

It takes a village to raise a child.
It also takes a village to care for an elder.

My hope is that every family caregiver at some point in the caregiving journey will come to grips with the fact that they *need* help and it is okay to *ask* for help. Caregivers do not need to endure the 24/7 grind of caring for a loved one on their own. For some, it takes much longer than for others to acknowledge this reality.

Ideally, many caregivers would like help to come in the form of another family member assisting and providing the care. When caring for a parent, the primary caregiver may believe if they are making the sacrifices, then surely their siblings should be willing to make sacrifices as well. After all, it's their mother or father too. In other cases, it's expected other relatives will see and understand the need and feel obliged to help out as well.

All too often, however, this isn't the case due to distance, other obligations and sometimes simply an inability or un-willingness to be a caregiver. Oftentimes, particularly among siblings, the caregiver tends to feel as though they're an only child caring for their parent because their siblings won't help out. Some siblings feel like they can't do what the primary caregiver does, and they're made to feel inadequate. They are not made to feel that *whatever* it is they can offer is helpful, needed and important.

When I mediate family discussions, I often ask family members to focus on what they are able to do. I ask them, "What *can* you bring to the table? What can we count on you to do? The primary caregiver needs your support and when you are not able to provide your time, your monetary contribution can assist in bringing in help to be there in your stead. Simply stated, it's either your time or your money that is needed." I would then encourage the primary caregiver to appreciate what's given, and to express their gratitude directly.

An Unintended Consequence

Because I moved my own mother away from her home to where I lived, I unwittingly created an unintended isolation for both of us. Many times I wanted siblings and other relatives to show up, but it was not practical or realistic. Those I thought would or should make it a priority to visit, see and care for my mom, couldn't or didn't. Some felt it was too hard to see Mom in her incapacitated state. I realized early on I needed help and I didn't hesitate to ask for it.

Sometimes when you cry for help, those you expect to answer, can't or won't. Sometimes you get an answer and it is not what you hope for or expect. The saving grace for me was that others did hear my cry for help. My sister-in-loves, Tina and Anya, were wonderful. So was my big sister, girlfriend, Pat, in providing regular support for Mom. Anya and Pat routinely traveled from Seattle and Las Vegas to help me care for Mom, providing coverage so I could travel for work or they could provide respite for my husband and me.

Each of them was invaluable and selfless in their dedication and assistance throughout our entire caregiving journey.

Tina, who oversaw and provided Mom's initial care when the pituitary brain tumor was discovered, stayed faithful and committed to supporting Mom. My mom's sisters visited and helped out when they could in the best way that they could.

I always had expectations that certain people would be there, simply because of who my mom was to them and how she had been such a giver her entire life. I eventually came to understand that *who* provided the help wasn't important. What mattered was the help needed was provided. I had to release the expectations I had of others and accept that my mother would have what she needed when she needed it.

As primary caregiver I had high and sometimes unrealistic standards for the professional caregivers who came in to care for my mother. I wanted them to do things as I did them. I needed them to engage my mother like *I* engaged her. At the time, I had no idea how ridiculous that expectation was.

Nobody could take care of my mom like I could, so what I thought I needed was a clone of me. Unintentionally, at times, I even made my own siblings feel inadequate when they would step in. We had rules, standards and conditions in place for my mother's wellbeing that had to be adhered to. Was that too much to ask? Clearly, it was.

The first extraordinary caregiver was my husband, Kevin. He had an incredible sense of love, respect and empathy for my mom. God, for sure, knew what He was doing when he made Kevin my husband. Kevin is a firefighter and has that special gene for caring about and being willing to sacrifice for others. When I was bone marrow exhausted, Kevin was there to insist I take care of myself. Then he would step in to take care of Mom. When I traveled, he oversaw Mom's care and did whatever needed to be done. My husband was so exceptional as a caregiver often times, to my dismay, Mom actually preferred him over me. Those who knew my mom best knew she was always, like her mom, just a wee bit partial to the men in her life, particularly her sons.

In the midst of our all encompassing experience as caregivers, I was keenly aware we were only five years into our marriage, yet our lives were consumed with caring for my mom. Mom required 24/7 care because of the stroke; everything but feeding had to be done for her. Balance in our lives was not available and I knew we had to find a way to create balance. This urgency was further enhanced as my husband's parents were aging and would soon require our attention as well. We needed to get this right, fast. Balance and sanity would be accomplished through creating a team that would provide the much needed additional help.

The agencies we worked with were encouraged to send us the best staff they could offer. We went through so many "professional" caregivers in the first eighteen months that I truly lost count. The process was both frustrating and exhausting.

In many instances the very basic skill set was lacking. In other instances, the basics were there but the caregiver simply didn't appear to care enough. It was clear this was nothing more than a "job" to them. We wanted and needed more. The hunt for quality care providers dragged on. It got to the point that asking for the right caregiver was my constant and most fervent prayer.

By the time Katryna came into our lives, I was a skeptic and pretty jaded. We had had a few very good caregivers but the best ones had been very limited in their availability due to the agency's low pay scale. Those caregivers could be counted on for weekend care, which we paid for out of pocket, giving my husband and me a bit of time for each other. However, Katryna would be available eight hours a day, five days a week. The cost for Mom's care was being covered by the Medicaid Long-Term Care/Home and Community Based Services Program. We had been approved for 40 hours per week. That was a monumental blessing to us.

At first, I focused on what Katryna couldn't do—skills she didn't have. She was from Russia and had a very heavy accent. If I had to strain to understand her English, how would she be able to communicate with my mom? Then there were the cultural differences. As a new immigrant, how would she be able to relate to my mom? Katryna was very close in age to me, so for that I was glad, but still, was she strong enough to transfer and lift mom?

Prayers Answered

As I complained about the shortcomings I perceived in this new prospect, the nurse case manager looked me square in the eyes and said, "She is the very best I have. If she's not good enough to meet your mom's needs, then I really don't have anyone who is." Her directness and firm tone of voice were just what I needed to snap me back to reality.

Somehow I managed to miss the crucial fact of Katryna being a "medical doctor." Katryna was studying for board exams so she could practice medicine in this country. She was a bonafide, dedicated professional who truly cared about her patients. I was narrow minded in my focus and nearly took a pass on her. I began to notice what was extraordinary about her rather than focusing on what was different. She was mature with a strong, solid nature. Her face was striking, but often understated. She never wanted to draw attention to herself. Katryna routinely pulled her brown hair back and wore her doctor's scrubs, underscoring her intentions and her purpose.

To say Katryna was an extraordinary professional caregiver would be an understatement. She would take care of my mother in a way that was different from mine but a way that was more than adequate and much better in some respects. Katryna saw my mother's needs from a different perspective. She allowed her to have a say and make her own decisions based on what she wanted as opposed to what we vehemently believed was best for Mom. Katryna's strong accent was soon lyrical to my ears and something we all came to love.

As for cultural differences, my entire family learned about Russian culture and I personally fell in love with Katryna's favorite Russian wine as we were all slowly introduced to a new and wonderful cuisine. We developed a penchant for Katryna's borscht, mini pies and dumplings. Katryna offered mom a friendship that I almost denied and an opportunity to learn about parts of the world that none of us had known about before.

We exposed Katryna to our culture as well. My heart smiled the day I walked in from work to find Mom asleep and Katryna singing along to Louis Armstrong's "Wonderful World" playing in the background. Katryna fell in love with all of the old, classic movies that my mom watched and became a fan of Sidney Poitier, Frank Sinatra and Sammy Davis, Jr.

Despite all of Mom's hospital stays and routine doctor visits, it would be Katryna who would first detect the lump on my mother's breast and best explain the course that my mother's illness would likely take. For the last 18 months of her life, my incredible mom had a medical doctor caring for her eight hours a day, five days a week. I came to see this miraculous circumstance as a divine gift in return for my mother's generosity to others over many years.

With Katryna on board, I could relax, take off my care-giver hat and resume being a daughter. I had been wearing that hat for so long I had lost my identity as my mother's daughter. I had been on automatic pilot as a caregiver for too long. In Katryna, Mom had an excellent doctor and caregiver forty hours a week. Katryna's help allowed Kevin and me to resume our roles as daughter and son-in-love. So even when Katryna wasn't there, we were able to be who Mom needed us to be first, and then we took care of her needs as caregivers. Becoming consumed with the role of caregiving is a pitfall that conscious caregivers must learn to avoid. Try as you may, you can never, ever be *all* things to your loved one.

Family caregivers often have a tough juggling act. As advocate and caregiver, it's easy to become so consumed with the role we forget how much, if not more so, we are needed in the relationship as son, daughter, spouse or friend. Those boundaries are easier to maintain if you have a support system of professional and family caregivers. Asking for and seeking help is essential to being able to provide the quality of care your loved one needs and the assistance you, as a caregiver, deserve to have.

So many of these stories emphasize help is available if it is asked for directly. Once help comes along, it is good for everyone if it is accepted for who gave it and the style in which it was given. The crucial ingredient in the process of caregiving is to express gratitude for the help that has been given. Acknowledgment is a powerful tool, blessing both the giver and the receiver. It is one of the unexpected gifts of the caregiving journey.

Teepa was Queen of the Thank You. She poured every ounce of gratitude her soul carried into every thank you she gave.

recipe card

Teamwork, It Works— 110 Pound Minimum

1. Stir in appreciation for the exceptional caregivers in your life. If they do an amazing job, tell them so, and *show* your appreciation.
2. Add as many family members to the recipe as possible. Ask everyone to support you. Let them know you need and want their help.
3. Remember, you are creating a delicious and healthy meal everyone will partake in. Don't expect family members or other caregivers to do things the way you do them. Everyone has their own ideas and ways of doing things, and that is OK. That's where the magic comes in. The combination of ingredients is key.
4. Simmer the idea that people want to help, but need the primary caregiver to let them know *how* to help. Keep a running list of "Things I need help with." When someone asks if there's anything they can do, grab the list and allow them to choose.

chapter ten

Gratitude

*No matter the season, we can all discover
there is much to be grateful for.*

We will never know if Teepa's choice to stay in her home after Will passed away was best for her or not. What I do know is it was definitely her wish, her desire to do so. At no point did she ever waver. Though not a viable option, she was more than willing to have any of her children or grandchildren move in with her.

Moving Teepa to Minnesota to live near her daughter was considered by the family, but the option never appealed to Teepa. It was always difficult for her adult children to know which decision was the right one. There were times when Teepa did fairly well with her circumstances, and other times when the mental and emotional strain of dealing with Will's loss seemed too much for her to bear. It helped when career opportunities relocated her grandson and his wife to the area. These were family members she could see on a regular basis, helping her feel less alone.

When adult children have to make decisions contrary to their parents' wishes, it can be an agonizing choice. All their lives they have looked up to their parents, respecting their decisions, believing their parents have always known what's best. It can be daunting when the time comes to make decisions on their behalf. Moving someone with dementia can be especially difficult. Taking them out of their familiar environment can cause a rapid decline in their mental state. When that decline happens while they are still in their own environment, knowing what to do and when to do it can create quite a dilemma.

My experience dictates that, as tough as it is, in many cases this role reversal must take place. There may come a time when parents need their adult children to determine what's best and make those hard choices, even when those choices are contrary to a parent's wishes. The questions must always begin by addressing their safety and what is in the parent's best interest.

A Legacy for Teepa

In Teepa's case, her children decided as long as the resources provided for the 24/7 care she required, they would allow Teepa to continue living in her home. Incredibly, that care ranged from $15,000 on the high end to $10,000 per month on the low end. Will saw to it those resources would be available, and the children carried out his wishes. There were so many days Teepa wanted one thing and one thing only, simply to be with her man, Will.

A remarkable characteristic of Teepa's was the depth of gratitude she always expressed to her caregivers. She was always grateful and appreciative for any and everything they did for her. I often heard her high pitched voice become just a bit louder as she said the most heartfelt and soul stirring,

"Thank you for everything." Her adult children were equally expressive of their appreciation to all of the caregivers and to me as well. They had evidently learned from their mother to take the time and energy to express gratitude in a powerful, gracious way.

Ellie was yet another caregiver who bonded with Teepa and connected quite effectively with her. One evening I got a routine call from Ellie asking if I would talk to Teepa. She had had a rather difficult evening and needed to be reassured.

When Teepa got on the phone she asked, "Nadine, did Will leave me for another woman?" Ellie and I assured her Will was and had always been blind when it came to other women. She had nothing to worry about.

There were days when Teepa's dementia would wreak havoc. She would often repeat herself and the caregivers would patiently redirect or answer the question again. She would also become highly agitated and it would be challenging to calm her down. Teepa's health overall was fair, but eventually the time came when Teepa's pacemaker needed to be replaced. We were all a bit nervous about her going under anesthesia, but she handled the procedure like a champ. It had been just over two years since Will's passing and though Teepa experienced rough patches, she was coping better than anyone expected.

A couple of weeks later her caregivers reported Teepa had lost consciousness for a brief moment while taking her shower. She was taken to the ER and was given a thorough check. There was an irregularity with the pacemaker and the follow-up plan called for another test of the new pacemaker.

It took a day to secure an appointment to see the cardiologist and another four days before she could be seen. I was livid as it appeared to me the medical office was not making it a priority to get her in to check the pacemaker. Teepa's son had to calm me down. On the day of her appointment, Teepa was given a very thorough examination by the cardiologist. The pacemaker was checked and it was determined it was functioning properly. He advised us there could be something wrong, but whatever it was, it wasn't the pacemaker and it wasn't her heart. It was the end of the day and the doctor arranged for Teepa to have a cat scan the next morning at the hospital. He thought it might be possible that Teepa had a blood clot in her leg.

When we wrapped up the appointment, I explained to Teepa I would be heading to Los Angeles on a late flight to see my 97-year-old grandmother. My grandmother wasn't doing well and she wanted to see me. I informed Teepa that the nurse and Angela, her caregiver, would be taking her to the appointment early the next morning. Teepa wished me well and gave me a great big hug. She said the most heartfelt and emphatic, "Thank you for everything."

I arrived in Los Angeles late that evening as scheduled. I went right to bed and awoke to the phone ringing at six a.m. It was Angela calling. When I said "Good morning," she said, "It's not a good morning. Teepa went to sleep but she didn't wake up."

I felt the tears springing to my eyes and immediately recalled the heartfelt thanks she had expressed just hours before, her warm hands entwining mine. Teepa had thanked me for everything I had done for her during the past three years as though she knew it would be her last chance to do so. Perhaps in her own way, Teepa had reached acceptance and surrender before I had. Certainly gratitude paves the way for achievement of these steps.

I now had the somber task of calling Teepa's oldest son to share this news. I apologized for the early call and then said, "Your Mom got her wish. Teepa is now back with her man." I instinctively framed her passing as the achievement of her deepest desire, my attempt to help all of us **accept** and **surrender** to the loss of this precious woman.

It was Memorial Day Weekend. I would spend time with my grandmother and other family members and head back to assist Teepa's family in planning her services. I couldn't help but feel a twinge of guilt that I wasn't there immediately to support the caregivers and Teepa's family. This loss impacted me in a way that was very different from the passing of other clients. After nearly three years of consulting and providing care management services to Will and Teepa, I didn't feel like a client had died; I felt like I had lost a member of my family. On reflection, I think it was being on call 24/7 and being so intrinsically involved in every aspect of Will and Teepa's lives that bonded me to them in a special sort of way. It was also their inherent goodness that allowed the three of us and their caregivers to share a really precious connection.

It turned out, the passing of Will and Teepa would be pivotal for me, leading to a shift in how I would conduct my business. As a professional, it's important to realize when you need to take a step back and re-assess. Seeking support to assist you in decompressing is routinely necessary. This case allowed me to bring my team of professionals, a licensed clinical social worker, a nurse and a gerontologist to assist in their care management. The team was exceptional but the time intensiveness of the case was extraordinary. Over the next few months, I made the decision to shift my focus from care management to caregiver coaching and consulting. This decision would allow me to support caregivers and extend my reach by serving more families in a direct and efficient manner.

I also came to understand that I had forgotten a very essential element in my work. I had become so serious that I had forgotten to laugh and find humor in my daily encounters. My own family was now providing 24/7 caregiving to our matriarch, my grandmother, and there was no shortage of opportunities to laugh heartily and often.

recipe card

Gratitude—
As Much As You Can Add

1. No matter what you're experiencing, there is always *something* to be grateful for.
2. If you think things are bad, a lack of gratitude can only make things worse.
3. Gratitude costs nothing. Stir in generously every day.
4. If you are a caregiver, express gratitude to your loved one for allowing you to serve them. Even if they can't express gratitude to you, appreciate the fact that you are in the position to care for them.
5. If you are a care recipient, no matter how difficult things may be for you, expressing gratitude to your caregivers for their love, support and caring is the daily gift they deserve and you can readily provide.
6. Garnish everything with gratitude and appreciation, and serve immediately.

chapter eleven

Funny Honey

We often times take ourselves too seriously.
Seek joy in the ordinary, look for reasons to smile, and
find a reason to laugh.

Some of us called her Lizzie Mae. Others called her Momma, Liz, Elizabeth, Granny or Grandmother. But I often referred to my mother's mom as Hurricane Lizzie (but never, ever to her face). All her life, Elizabeth Harrell St. Cyr had indeed been a force to be reckoned with. She was only 4'8" tall, a stony, petite, powerful little woman that no one in their right mind would ever mess with. You could see the force coming from her in her forward leaning stance, her sharp nose, strong chin, and the bony hand that grasped her gold handled cane.

Elizabeth—Hurricane Lizzie—was a very stern, but protective mother and grandmother. She ruled with a firm hand, a baseball bat and a broomstick, commanding respect from everyone who came in contact with her. She was a strong disciplinarian, a woman of fierce conviction. When she said something, you best believe she meant what she said and said what she meant. She never tolerated *any* disrespect. She had no problems correcting anyone. My grandmother was honest and would tell you the truth whether you wanted to hear it or not. A lie, she would never tell. And though she was stern, she was also nurturing, had a listening ear and kept her house full of love and laughter. Besides that, she had style. For her 90th birthday, she organized us all into outfits that were color coordinated with hers—a black chiffon dress accented by a red beaded necklace and belt.

My fondest memory of Momma was she was an outstanding cook and would make ordinary food taste divine. She could make shrimp and okra stew so good the aroma would have you salivating. The sautéed shrimp and ham along with onions, bell peppers and garlic marinating in tomato sauce, served over a mound of rice was spectacular, and one of my all-time favorite dishes. It was my grandmother who was the queen of gumbo and taught my mother and all of her sisters everything she knew about it. Gumbo at my grandparents' home was a special occasion everyone looked forward to.

It was Labor Day Weekend, September 2013. I headed to Los Angeles to visit her for what I thought would be the final time. Warm and fuzzy isn't what I ever got from my grandmother, and this trip would be no exception. At 97, she was tired, in a lot of pain, and refusing all meds that might make her feel better. She was eating little or nothing and drinking very little. She would barely take a sip of gumbo. She had never been sick, but her diagnosis was failure to thrive. Anything else she might have had, we wouldn't know because she refused to go the doctor. Even with dementia, at 97 years of age she was impressively sharp, though occasionally confused.

I often explain to clients that dementia can either alter the personality or enhance the personality. In my grandmother's case, her personality was enhanced and magnified. Always strong and quite opinionated, on this visit, she was absolutely cantankerous and downright mean. For me, this was hard to take. As one of her oldest and most favored grandchildren, I had been spared Lizzie's wrath, but now I was experiencing it firsthand.

My grandmother now had a salty response for any and everything that was said to her.

As we begged and cajoled her to eat and brought food to her, her response would be, "Get that crap outta my face. I'm not eating that."

If we asked what she wanted to eat, she might or might not respond. On rare occasion she would tell you what she wanted, you would bring her that very food, and then she would say, "I didn't ask for it. I do not want it and I will not eat it!"

During that visit, when her mood had shifted a bit, I asked if she remembered how to make her shrimp and okra stew. She told me she didn't remember. I was certain if I got the ingredients, together we would figure it out. I did just that and when preparation time came, she shared all she could remember. I made a huge pot of her famous shrimp and okra stew and everyone loved it. My grandmother, however, refused to taste a single bite.

Momma lived with her younger daughter, my Aunt Bev and her daughters, Dani and Tee. They were her three primary caregivers. Aunt Bev is tall and striking in posture and demeanor. She has the medium build that most of my grandfather's children possess. Aunt Bev is the type you can hardly ever upset. She will find a reason to laugh at anything. I marveled at how nothing my grandmother ever said or did seemed to faze my Aunt Bev. She would just laugh when my grandmother said outlandish things. She was concerned if Momma didn't eat, but she simply found a way to not let it get to her. I would often ask Aunt Bev how she was coping with things. She said, "I do what I can do. I do what she allows me to and the rest I just can't worry about. And after that, I laugh about it."

Diva Dani is a teacher, gorgeous, inside and out and very much a fashionista. My cousin Dani was the quiet sweetheart that Momma adored, most of the time. When all else failed, Dani would be called in to cajole Momma and sometimes get her to do what was needed.

Last but not least was Tee, good looking in a short and stocky way. Cousin Tee was a comedian in her own right. She would don one of our grandmother's house dresses, put on a wig and imitate my grandmother so well we would all laugh until we cried. Tee, however, was quite concerned about her own mother, Aunt Bev, and the toll that 24/7 caregiving was having on her. Tee dearly loved our grandmother, but she was fiercely protective of her mom. She insisted her mom take breaks and facilitated getting as many family members as possible involved in taking care of our grandmother. My cousin innately understood the necessity of the team approach to caregiving.

Tee and our grandmother had a rather special relationship. Momma would pretend to be mad at her but would find herself snickering at something she would say. Being one of the family historians, Tee would try to get our grandmother to provide information about her history. Most of the time, Momma just wasn't telling, but on rare occasion, Tee could get her to open up and share. On one occasion Momma told her about a gun she had taken from her grandson that she still had. Nobody believed that wild story and blamed it on the dementia. Tee, however, did believe her. More importantly, if she had a gun, Tee was motivated to find it because Momma's behavior was such that she might get mad enough and use that gun on any one of us!

Family as a Team

Getting help from family members on a regular and consistent basis was challenging at first, but eventually everyone settled into a routine of helping out and pitching in as the caregiver's third step, **process,** was achieved. My uncles would visit their mom routinely and my aunts were vigilant in assisting Aunt Bev by pulling their share of the weight in caring for their mother.

One of the biggest challenges for all of my grandmother's children was the role reversal that must sometimes take place between adult children and their parents. Because my grandmother had always ruled with an iron fist, the idea of making the tough decisions which needed to be made on her behalf was challenging at best. Even with dementia, my grandmother was never willing to relinquish decision making to anyone. When she said she didn't want to do something, nothing anyone said or did could change her mind. When an ambulance was called to take her to the emergency room, she vehemently refused and threatened the paramedics. They said they could not take her to the hospital if she did not want to go, and she did not go.

Grumpy though she was, I had a deep need to be with my grandmother, so I traveled back and forth to Los Angeles several times before she passed. On my final visit in December, prior to my arrival, she had been semi-conscious for a few days. When I arrived she woke up, knew who I was, and was genuinely glad to see me. She asked, "Hey Na, when did you get here?" I was surprised by her alertness and her reaction to me. But I was also startled by how emaciated my grandmother had become. Later in the day, she was sitting up in bed and said she wanted fried catfish so off Aunt Bev and I ran to get it. Though she couldn't eat it, it gave us satisfaction just knowing she wanted it.

The Final Visit

My grandmother had mystified hospice for months because on a number of occasions the staff thought it was only a matter of time and she likely wouldn't make it through the night. On the third day of the final visit I got out of the house for an overdue massage and ran a few errands. That night I figured I'd sit up with the nurse and hold vigil while my aunts got some rest.

The nurse said Momma's vitals were strong, she was resting peacefully, and I should get some rest because my grandmother was just fine. I just had this feeling I needed to stay by her side. Together, the hospice nurse and I prayed over my grandmother. Following prayer, I simply talked to Momma, told her how much we all loved her, and knew it was time for her to go. I assured her we would all be okay. Sometimes the caregiver's **acceptance** of the impending loss of their loved one needs to be expressed to them. This permission to leave helps the dying person **surrender** to their own passing.

I told Momma all the things I wanted her to tell my mom who was already up there waiting for her. Then I reminded her that Grandpa, Uncle Butz, Aunt Janie, Betty and Olivia, Tony and Arthur, and of course her parents, siblings, and a whole bunch of other folk were all waiting for her in heaven.

It dawned on me then why I needed to be with my grandmother. Momma had been right there with me five years earlier as we said goodbye to my mom, her oldest daughter. It was only fitting that I would have the privilege to be with my mother's mother as she made her transition.

Tee and her girlfriend, Leslie, came in the room at that moment and were overcome with emotion and couldn't stay. I began to sing "I Shall Wear a Crown," and Hurricane Lizzie, very quietly, left to join my grandfather, my mom and the rest of the family serving as her welcoming committee.

My grandmother passed on an indelible legacy. She and my grandfather, Edmond, took seriously and literally the scripture, "Be fruitful and multiply." They had 12 children, 39 grandchildren, 61 great grandchildren and 42 great, great grandchildren. The family tree continues to grow from 154 to who knows how many. We are an amazing, crazy, very loud, fun-loving and sometimes functional family.

More than a year after my grandmother's death, Tee and Aunt Bev were in the backyard, clearing out my grandmother's belongings, some of which had been placed in the shed. And there it was. Right there, behind two boxes, stuffed in a hat box and wrapped in a grey towel, was the Smith & Wesson with a pearl white handle. It was the very gun my grandmother told Tee about. Hurricane Lizzie did not tell a lie. Aunt Bev and Tee both screamed and ran when they realized what they had found. They had another good laugh but not until after they contacted authorities to remove the gun. They were both too chicken to even touch that gun.

I sometimes take for granted the gift of family that I am blessed to have. A small family gathering for us typically consists of at least thirty people. An average gathering will draw fifty family members. With that comes a lot of joy. Over the past several years, we've come to understand the one, major downside of a large family is that you eventually lose loved ones to illness and death. In the past decade alone, we have lost ten relatives from the St. Cyr family tree. It got to the place where we were primarily seeing each other at funerals and we decided we would change that.

Now, cousins' reunions are held. We even take vacations together and gather for major birthdays and anniversaries, weddings and retirement parties. Next year, we'll be trying a first, a family cruise with one hundred of us taking over the friendly seas.

Our family has changed. My mother and my grandparents are no longer physically with us. My grandfather was the core and rock of our family. My grandmother was the first caregiver I knew. She cared for family members because it was simply what she knew to do. Caring for others was second nature to her. My mother, her oldest daughter, possessed a loving nature and was a caring person her entire life. The baton was passed to me. I have dropped it on an occasion or two but have strived to assist and support others along this journey to accept the role of caregiving in the manner that best suits them. I hope to encourage others to do so, not out of guilt or responsibility, but from the understanding that caring for others is an honor. Whether we are conscious of it or not, Anam Cara lives within each one of us. This Celtic concept of the divinity of the caregiving experience is typified in those caregivers who hold nothing back from the experience.

recipe card
Funny Honey—1 Gallon

1. There will be days when your loved one will make Gus cuss. Laugh out loud!
2. Don't take yourself so seriously.
3. Free will is the last thing that your loved one has to hold onto. Respect and honor their wishes. If they don't thank you for your efforts, don't sulk—find something to laugh about!
4. You cannot change the course of disease in someone else's body. All you can do is learn as much as you can, do what you're allowed to do and respect the wishes of your loved one.
5. This is their journey. You are simply a passenger along for the ride.
6. Hospice is a great resource and a most valuable asset for caregivers and their loved ones.
7. Hospice improves your loved one's quality of life as well as the family's quality of life.
8. When your loved one no longer wants to eat, respect that. Dying is hard work and the body no longer needs food, nor can it process it.
9. Death is the final frontier for all of us. Get over your fear and recognize that nothing any of us do will allow us to escape the inevitable.
10. Bring to a rolling boil. Nobody's getting out of here alive!

chapter twelve

Anam Cara,
Carer of the Soul

*The soul-to-soul connection that happens between the
caregiver and care recipient is the evidence of God.*

The lessons that I have learned as caregiver and consultant
are innumerable. The experiences I have shared and the
beautiful people I have been blessed to know have been gifts
like no other.

As I accepted the assignment I was given to become a
Caregiver Consultant, Care Manager and Caregiver Coach,
I knew education was critical. I learned a lot from fifteen
years of caring for my mom, but I needed to learn much more.
I volunteered and trained with the Alzheimer's Association
and learned all I could about dementia and its impact on the
family. I earned a Professional Advancement Gerontology
Certification from the University of Colorado Gerontology
Center. I earned a Certification as a Senior Advisor (CSA)
and Patient Navigator. I obtained training in Medicaid and
Medicare so I could assist caregivers in multiple arenas.

I also knew enough to know that I still needed additional
resources and individuals on my team. I contracted with

JoKatherine Holliman Page, LCSW and Rodella Wooten, LCSW, as well as Gerontologist, Terri Howard. To complete the tribe, we added Dr. Na Notchka Chumley to our team. They are all dedicated, heart centered professionals who know the caregiving journey and who enhance the work that we do at TCG. With all of that, there was still a key ingredient that was needed.

Spiritual training is, has been and will be one of the most valuable facets of this learning process. I have been honored to know people of different faiths and walks of life where each has their own viable and real connection to God. To further facilitate my own personal growth, I participated in the *What Will Set You Free Training* offered by Cynthia James Enterprises and was certified as a Freedom Coach. Two years of training and practice provided a vital, necessary spiritual tool in anchoring me and assisting my caregivers on their journeys.

Anam Cara Within

One of the profound discoveries I made along this journey was of the *Anam Cara*. This is a Celtic phrase which means Carer of the Soul. I have been blessed to work with many caregivers and professionals who are indeed *Anam Cara*. That powerful but vulnerable bond speaks from the care recipient saying, "You are the physical spirit that I trust to care for me and escort me along this journey as I move from this realm to the next."

In reply, the caregiver or *Anam Cara* gently whispers, "It is my honor. Thank you for choosing me."

The caregivers who travel this sometimes arduous, often difficult, seemingly impossible journey can and may well encounter grace and eventually recognize the *Anam Cara* within. Those who do will understand the greater good and higher purpose they have been called to serve.

Anam Cara is exemplified in some form in every story in this book. I certainly carried my mother's soul, with lots of help, through her fifteen-year series of medical issues. I may have started my journey in resistance, but with the example of Miss Yvonne, I learned how to devote myself to this task and to reap the reward of intimacy and love like no other. I have been blessed by the honor of *Anam Cara* every day of my life since my mother passed.

Miss Yvonne was competent in every aspect of her life, and her ability to serve as *Anam Cara* for her mother and brother was part of her inherent savvy. She knew how to serve them, how to get help and support, and how to care for herself, all at the same time. Her stance, now that she is alone, is victorious. It has been the honor of her life to serve her beloveds as their *Anam Cara*.

Heroic Will did everything he knew to do as *Anam Cara* for his darling Teepa. If he had not been such a strong and stubborn man, he might have known to reach out for help sooner. In this circumstance, his children sensed the liability in his heroism and made efforts to bring help into the lives of their parents. I hope they see themselves as *Anam Caras* for their beloved parents, even though they were not 24/7 caregivers for them.

Among all these caregivers, it is Dahlia who was most prepared and ready to serve as *Anam Cara* for her mother. Because she was already deeply established in a spiritual journey, the steps of **acceptance** and **surrender** were open doors for her. She and her daughter, Janie, continue to take care of Sarah who is maintaining a peaceful existence. And why wouldn't she? She is living in The House of Grace, after all. There is no angst around the fact that Sarah hasn't left yet. The house is at peace. When it comes time to accept her mother's passing, Dahlia will do so with grace.

Hurricane Lizzie, the matriarch of my family, was larger than life. It is no surprise that many of her daughters, sons and granddaughters were blessed to serve as *Anam Cara* for her. She created a tribe, and they were honored to serve her during her time of illness. In companioning my grandmother in her final hour of life as she joined my mother and grandfather, I was blessed again with surrender, a surrender which reverberated from my grandmother to my mother, from the present death to the previous one. In being there for that moment, I was honored beyond all honor, healed, and redeemed.

Some of us willingly answer the call to be a caregiver while others do so dodging, kicking and screaming. It does not matter what category you fall into, you have the capacity to make that all-important connection, to honor life, love and relationship in such a way that when the journey ends, there is a peace that surpasses all understanding. We come to realize the goal, for ourselves and our loved ones, ultimately is about surrender, creating soul content.

I would like to underscore the broad nature of the term *Anam Cara* as it applies to caregivers. It is not just a concept which operates between a parent and child, or a husband and wife. *Anam Cara* lives between any two people who help each other along the journey of life. The Carer of the Soul or Soul Friend is present when a friend supports another going through a time of distress. With or without the label, the relationship exists. The blessing of the label is it allows the caregiver to accept and honor what they are doing.

The Soul Connection

All great chefs know that a recipe is merely a guide to the creation of a spectacular dish. Chefs also know that using their sixth sense to enhance a recipe is often necessary. The recipe is merely a suggestion for creating the base of a dish. It's the chef's special touch, a sense of knowing, that ultimately makes a good dish a great dish.

As a caregiver, you know your loved one better than anyone. You know what works for them and what doesn't. You know when something is off with them no matter what the medical professionals say. You understand their reactions to medications and environment. They are dependent upon you to make the best choices for them and you are equipped to do that, even if you think you aren't. So use the recipes in this book as a guide. Make adjustments to the recipe steps and ingredients based on your loved one's needs and your sense of knowing. Take time to assess, tap into and trust your sixth sense.

Just like making gumbo, there isn't anything clear about making the caregiving journey.

- It is complex, multi-faceted, often times messy, and things can sometimes get heated.
- It's a hodgepodge of feelings, emotions, highs and lows, good intentions and a flurry of activities that are best done in community.
- It has mysterious ingredients, a number of variables and spices that can slowly but eventually come

together to create a symphony of goodness that feeds the soul.

- It is patience and gratitude that brings you to the simmering point of soul contentment, which fills and nourishes you, bringing peace, joy and eventually understanding.

The caregiver's journey can be just like a great big delicious bowl of my grandmother's, my mom's and now *my* Louisiana Seafood Gumbo if it is tended to in community, with care and love.

recipe card

Anam Cara, Carer of the Soul— Season to Taste

1. Learn all you can about your loved one's illness and their prognosis.
2. Develop a daily spiritual practice that will support you on this journey.
3. You are a caregiver. Be proud of it.
4. It is an honor to be of service. Be present and embrace that truth.
5. Place your role as caregiver in perspective. Be the caregiver you would want to have.
6. An *Anam Cara* is a Carer of the Soul. There is *no* greater honor than to care for a loved one as they begin their transition.
7. Bask in the joy of knowing you have made an incredible difference.
8. Be proud of yourself for what you have been able to do.
9. Forgive yourself for what you could not do.
10. There is meaning and purpose in your journey. Sooner or later, it will be revealed, and you will indeed be healed, restored and redeemed.

Glossary

Activities of Daily Living (ADL's): Assessment which measures the functional status of a person. **Basic ADLs** are fundamental self-care tasks that include personal hygiene and grooming, dressing and undressing, feeding, transferring—moving on and off of a chair or bed—and toileting. **Instrumental ADLs** are not necessary for fundamental functioning, but they allow an individual to continue to live independently. These include housework and shopping for groceries, meal preparation, taking medications, managing money and use of a telephone.

Acute Care: Care that is generally provided for a short period of time to treat a certain illness or condition. This type of care can include short-term hospital stays.

Acute Illness: Illness that is usually short-term and that often comes on quickly.

Acute Pain: Pain that has a known cause and occurs for a limited time.

Adult Care Home: Also called board and care home or group home, an adult care home is a residence that offers housing and personal care services, such as meals, supervision, and transportation for residents.

Adult Day Care: Community-based care designed to meet the needs of impaired adults who, for their own safety and well-being, can no longer be left at home alone during the day. Offers much needed respite for the caregiver.

Administration on Aging (AOA): An agency of the U.S. Department of Health and Human Services that is the focal point for older persons and their concerns at the federal level.

Advance Medical Directives: Prepared ahead of time, a health care advance directive is a written document that states how a person wants medical decisions to be made if he or she loses the ability to make these decisions. A health care advance directive may include a Living Will, a Durable Power of Attorney for Health Care or both.

Advocate: A champion of caregivers, a supporter, promoter, one who speaks publicly on behalf of the care recipient.

Altered Mental Status: A disruption in how the brain works that causes a change in behavior. This change can happen suddenly or over days. AMS ranges from slight confusion to total disorientation and increased sleepiness to coma.

Alzheimer's Disease: Alzheimer's is a progressive brain disorder that destroys brain cells. Alzheimer's is not a normal part of aging. Alzheimer's is the most common type of dementia accounting for 60 to 80% of dementia cases. Some of the warning signs are forgetfulness severe enough to affect work, lifelong hobbies or social life, confusion, trouble planning and expressing thoughts, misplacing things, getting lost in familiar places, changes in personality or behavior

Ambulatory: Able to walk about.

Ambulatory with Assistance: Able to get about with the aid of a cane, crutch, brace, wheelchair or walker.

Ambulatory Care: All types of health services that are provided on an outpatient basis, instead of services provided in the home or to persons in a clinical setting.

Anam Cara: Carer of the Soul, Soul Friend.

Anticipatory Grief: Refers to a grief reaction that occurs before an impending loss. Typically, the impending loss is a death of someone close due to illness but it can also be experienced by dying individuals themselves.

Area Agency on Aging (AAA): A nationwide network of state and local programs that help older people plan and care for their life-long needs.

Assessment: Activities performed by at least one professional (preferably a social worker and/or a nurse) to determine a person's current ability to function in six areas: physical health, mental health, social support, activities of daily living, environmental conditions, and financial situation.

Assisted Living Facility (ALF): Residences that provide a "home with services" and that emphasize residents' privacy and choice. Assisted living residence means any group housing and services program for two or more unrelated adults that makes available, at a minimum, one meal a day and housekeeping services and provides personal care services to the residents. Settings in which services are delivered may include self-contained apartment units or single or shared room units with private or area baths.

Assistive Devices: A range of products designed to help seniors or people with disabilities lead more independent lives. Examples include motorized wheelchairs, walking aids, elevated toilet seats, bathtub seats, and handrails.

Autonomy: Making independent decisions or choices.

Anxiety: A feeling of worry, nervousness, or unease, typically about an imminent event or something with an uncertain outcome.

Bereavement: A period of mourning after a loss.

Boundaries: Guidelines, rules or limits that a caregiver creates to identify for themselves what are reasonable, safe and permissible ways for the care recipient to behave towards him or her and how they will respond when someone steps past those limits. Consciously determining what your capacity is as a caregiver.

Bone Marrow Exhaustion: Completely spent, mentally, physically and emotionally, typically experienced by caregivers who provide 24/7 care for a long period of time

Burden: The impact or consequence of having the responsibility of caring for someone who requires extensive care and is reliant upon the caregiver.

Burnout: Physical or mental collapse caused by overwork, caregiver exhaustion.

Care Management: Care management is a set of activities intended to improve patient care and reduce the need for medical services by helping patients and caregivers more effectively manage health conditions.

Care Plan: A written action plan that contains strategies for delivering care to address an individual's needs and problems.

Care Recipient: The person receiving care who typically has a condition such as Parkinson's disease, cancer, Alzheimer's disease, traumatic brain injury, AIDS, muscular dystrophy, paralysis, multiple sclerosis, frailty attributed to old age, or other chronic illness.

Caregiver: An adult who provides unpaid care for the physical and emotional needs of a family member or friend.

Caregiver Coaching: Customized service that equips family caregivers with knowledge, skills and tools to achieve a balanced lifestyle while caring for another.

Celebration of Life Event: An occasion to celebrate someone's life while they are present or a celebration in lieu of a traditional funeral. It can be individualized, unique and creative to best represent the honoree.

Certified: A long-term care facility, home health agency, or hospice agency that meets the requirements imposed by Medicare and Medicaid is said to be certified. Being certified is not the same as being accredited. Medicare, Medicaid and some long-term care insurance policies only cover care in a certified facility or provided by a certified agency.

Chronic Illness: An illness or other condition with one or more of the following characteristics: permanency, residual disability, requires rehabilitation training, or requires a long period of supervision, observation, or care. Typically, it is a disease or condition that lasts over a long period of time and cannot be cured; it is often associated with disability.

Chronic Pain: Pain that occurs for more than one month after healing of an injury, or that occurs repeatedly over months or that is due to a lesion that is not expected to heal.

Circle of Care: A team or support system that assists the caregiver with duties tasks or provides respite for the caregiver.

Clinical Trials: Carefully planned and monitored experiments to test a new drug or treatment.

Codicil: A written amendment to a will.

Collaborative care: A healthcare philosophy and movement that has many names, models, and definitions that often include the provision of mental health, behavioral health and substance use services in primary care.

Comfort Food: Food that provides consolation, a feeling of wellbeing, often associated with childhood, fond memories of a loved one and home.

Comprehensive: A full range of available services including various levels of nursing care, support therapies, psycho/social assessments, treatment and referral to appropriate resources.

Competence: Usually used in a legal sense, refers to a person's ability to understand information, make an informed choice based on the information and values, and communicate that decision.

Conservator: A court appointed guardian or a protector who is appointed by a judge to manage the financial affairs and/or daily life of another due to physical or mental limitations or old age.

Continence: The ability to maintain control of bowel and bladder function. Or, when unable to maintain control of these functions, the ability to perform associated personal hygiene (including caring for catheter or colostomy bag).

Continuing Care Retirement Community (CCRC): A retirement community that offers a broad range of services and levels of care based on what each resident needs over time. Sometimes called "life care," it can range from independent living in an apartment to assisted living to full-time care in a nursing home.

Continuum of Care: Encompasses the different care services considered necessary over the full course of an illness.

Co-Existing Illness: A medical condition or illness that occurs simultaneously with another and may complicate or obscure diagnosis or treatment of each.

Co-Payment: The specified portion that Medicare, health insurance, or a service program may require a person to pay toward his or her medical bills or services.

Covered Benefit or Service: A health service or item that is included in an insurance plan or policy, and that is paid for either partially or fully.

Covered Charge: Services or benefits for which a health plan makes either partial or full payment.

Cues: Both verbal and non-verbal prompts, instructions and gestures that assist persons in their daily living.

Custodial Care: Care to help individuals meet personal needs such as bathing, dressing, eating, and other non-medical care that most people do themselves, such as using eye drops. Medicare does not pay for custodial care and Medicaid pays very little.

Dehydration: Lack of adequate fluid in the body, a crucial factor in the health of older people.

Delirium: A disturbance of brain function that causes confusion and changes in alertness, attention, thinking and reasoning, memory, emotions, sleeping patterns and coordination. These symptoms may start suddenly, may be due to some type of medical problem, and may get worse or better multiple times.

Dementia: A general term for a group of brain disorders that cause mental decline severe enough to interfere with usual activities and daily life; affects more than one of the four core mental abilities: the ability to learn and recall new information; the ability to write or speak or to understand written or spoken words; the ability to understand and use symbols and maps; the ability to plan, reason, problem solve and focus on a task.

Denial: The refusal to admit the truth or reality or an inability to see the truth.

Directives: An order of instruction, i.e. advanced medical directive.

Disorientation: Loss of one's bearings, loss of sense of familiarity with one's surroundings, or loss of one's bearings with respect to time, place and person.

Do-Not-Resuscitate (DNR) Orders: Instructions written by a doctor telling other healthcare providers not to try to restart a patient's heart using cardiopulmonary resuscitation (CPR) or other related treatments if his/her heart stops beating. Usually, DNR orders are written after a discussion between a doctor and the patient and/or family members.

Durable Power of Attorney for Health Care (DPOAHC): A legal document that specifies one or more individuals (called a health care proxy) designated to make medical decisions for a person if that person is incapacitated.

End of Life Care: refers to health care, not only of patients in the final hours or days of their lives, but more broadly care of all those with a terminal illness or terminal disease condition that has become advanced, progressive and incurable.

Entitlement: Federal program (such as Social Security or unemployment benefits) that guarantees a certain level of benefits to those who meet requirements set by law.

Estate Planning: Thoughtful consideration and planning for an individual's future in the area of finances and property. In some cases, planning for health care decisions may begin at this time.

Extended Care: Short-term or temporary care in a hospital available for those awaiting permanent nursing home or less intense nursing care prior to returning home. The process of restoration of skills by a person who has had an illness or injury so as to regain maximum self-sufficiency and function in a normal or as near normal manner as possible.

Family Caregiver: Anyone who provides care without pay and who usually has personal ties to the care recipient. This person can provide full or part time help, and may live with the care recipient or separately.

Fiscal Intermediaries: Private insurance organizations under contract with the federal government to handle Medicare claims from hospitals, skilled nursing facilities and home health agencies (Part A).

Five Stages of Grief: Author Elizabeth Kubler Ross identified the stages as denial, anger, bargaining, depression and acceptance.

Five Steps of Conscious Caregiving: Author Nadine Roberts Cornish identified the stages as helplessness, recognition, process, acceptance and surrender.

Functional Status/Capabilities: The measurement (usually through a scale or instrument of assessment) of a person's abilities in activities of daily living or instrumental activities of daily living.

Geriatric Care Manager: Also known as "Aging Life Care™," "elder care management," "senior health care management" and "professional care management," is the process of planning and coordinating care of the elderly and others with physical and/or mental impairments to meet their long-term care needs, improve their quality of life, and maintain their independence for as long as possible. It entails working with persons of old age and their families in managing, rendering and referring various types of health and social care services.

Guardian: A legal term for a person who is lawfully vested with the care of a person who has been judged legally incompetent and/or the care of the person's property.

Health Care Proxy/Agent: A document (legal instrument) with which a patient appoints an agent to legally make healthcare decisions on behalf of the patient when he or she is incapable of making and executing the healthcare decisions stipulated in the proxy.

Health Maintenance Organization (HMO): An organization that, for a prepaid fee, provides a comprehensive range of health maintenance and treatment services (including hospitalization, preventive care, diagnosis, and nursing). HMOs are sponsored by large employers, labor unions, medical schools, hospitals, medical clinics, and insurance companies.

Home Health Agency (HHA): A public or private agency certified by Medicare that specializes in providing skilled nurses, homemakers, home health aides, and therapeutic services such as physical therapy in an individual's home.

Home Health Care: Health services provided in the homes of the elderly, disabled, sick, or convalescent. The types of services provided include nursing care, social services, home health aide and homemaking services, and various rehabilitation therapies (e.g., speech, physical and occupational therapy).

Hospice: A special way of caring for people with terminal illnesses and their families by keeping the patient as comfortable as possible by relieving pain and other symptoms, preparing for a death that follows the wishes and needs of the patient, and reassuring both the patient and family members by helping them to understand and manage what is happening.

Hospice Home Care: Most hospice patients receive care while living in their homes. Home hospice patients have family members or friends who provide most of their care, with help and support from the trained hospice team, which visits the house to provide medical and nursing care, emotional support, counseling, information, instruction, and practical help.

Incontinence: The loss of bowel and bladder control.

Informed Consent: The process of making decisions about medical care that are based on open, honest communication between the health care provider and the patient and/or the patient's family members.

Infusion Therapy: Injection of a solution directly into a vein.

Instrumental Activities of Daily Living (IADLs): Personal tasks often performed by a caregiver, such as meal preparation, grocery shopping, making telephone calls, and money management.

Interim Care: Same as "Extended Care."

Intermediate Care: Assistance with activities of daily living plus rehabilitation services usually provided by licensed therapists and registered nurses as well as licensed practical nurses.

Intermittent Care: A requirement for services to be covered by Medicare; home health services given to a patient at least once every 60 days or as frequently as a few hours a day, several times per week.

Licensed Practical Nurse (LPN): One who has completed one or two years in a school of nursing or vocational training school. LPNs are in charge of nursing in the absence of a Registered Nurse (RN). LPNs often give medications and perform treatments. They are licensed by the state in which they work.

Live-In: A person who will live in the home of an individual requiring health care to provide assistance to the individual.

Living Will: A legal document that outlines the kinds of medical care a patient wants and doesn't want. The living will is used only if the patient becomes unable to make decisions for him/herself.

Long Distance Caregiving: Typically a family member who lives 100 miles away from the care recipient and manages their financial affairs and medical needs.

Long-Term Care and Support: Refers to a broad and highly variable range of rehabilitative, restorative and health maintenance services that assist people with ADLs, IADLs and the emotional aspects of coping with illness or disability.

Long-Term Care Insurance (LTC): Coverage that provides nursing-home care, home-health care, personal or adult day care for individuals above the age of 65 or with a chronic or disabling condition who need constant supervision and have deficits in at least two of their activities of daily living.

Medicaid: An assistance program through which the federal government and the individual states share in payment for the medical care of certain categories of needy and low-income people.

Medicare: A federal health insurance program for people 65 and over and some under 65 who are disabled. Medicare has two parts. Part A is also called Hospital Insurance, and Part B is called Medical Insurance.

Medigap Insurance: Sold by private insurance companies, this type of insurance is specifically designed to help pay health care expenses either not covered or not fully covered by Medicare.

Meditate: To think deeply or focus one's mind for a period of time in silence or with the aid of chanting, for religious or spiritual purposes or as a method of relaxation.

Meditation: The action or process or meditating

Multi-Disciplinary Team/Interdisciplinary Team: A group of professionals with different skills and training who share information and consultation around a person's care.

Nursing Home: An institutional setting that offers 24-hour supervision and care to individuals, usually older persons, who are no longer able to be responsible for themselves in an independent living setting.

Nutrition/Hydration: Intravenous (IV) fluid and nutritional supplements given to patients who are unable to eat or drink by mouth, or those who are dehydrated or malnourished.

Occupational Rehabilitation Services (ORS): A program for persons under age 60 who are at risk of nursing home placement or who require information and assistance.

Ombudsman: A person who investigates complaints and assists in resolving problems that may arise in a long-term care facility.

Palliative Care: The total care of patients with progressive, incurable illness. In palliative care, the focus of care is on quality of life. Control of pain and other physical symptoms, and psychological, social and spiritual problems are considered most important.

Personal Care: Activities such as bathing, dressing, grooming, caring for hair/nails and oral hygiene needed to facilitate treatment or to prevent deterioration of a person's health.

Pharmacotherapy: The treatment of diseases and symptoms with medications.

Prognosis: A prediction of the probable course of a disease in an individual and the chances of recovery.

Prayer: A solemn expression of thanks, a request or petition in earnest addressed to God.

Registered Nurse (RN): A graduate nurse who has completed a minimum of two years of education at an accredited school of nursing. RNs are licensed by the state in which they work.

Rehabilitation: The process of restoration of skills by a person who has had an illness or injury so as to regain maximum self-sufficiency and function in a normal or as near normal manner as possible.

Reimbursement: Financial repayment for costs incurred by individuals in the care of a loved one.

Resilience: The power or ability to recover from difficulties.

Respite: Temporary or short-term care of a chronically ill person by another which is designed to give the caregiver a rest.

Ritual: Done as part of a ceremony or practice, typically done the same way each time.

Self-Care: Includes any intentional actions taken to care for one's physical, mental and emotional health. Self-care *must* be a priority for all caregivers.

Senility: Popularized laymen's term used by doctors and the public alike to categorize the mental deterioration that may occur with aging.

Senior Center: A community facility for senior citizens. Senior centers provide a variety of activities for their members, including a combination of recreational, educational, cultural, or social events. Also, some centers offer nutritious meals and limited health care services.

Skilled Care: A type of health care given when the patient needs skilled nursing or rehabilitation staff to manage, observe, and evaluate their care. Nursing, physical therapy, occupational therapy, and speech therapy are considered skilled care by Medicare. It may be administered in a Skilled Care Facility or at home.

Skilled Nursing Facility (SNF): A facility that has been certified by Medicare and/or Medicaid to provide skilled care.

Sleep Deprivation: The condition of not having enough sleep; it can be either chronic or acute. A chronic sleep-restricted state can cause fatigue, daytime sleepiness, clumsiness and weight loss or weight gain. It adversely affects the brain and cognitive function.

Social Security: A national insurance program that provides income to workers when they retire or are disabled and to dependent survivors when a worker dies. Retirement payments are based on worker's earnings during employment.

Social Worker: A person trained to identify social and emotional needs and provide services necessary to meet them.

Spend Down: Under the Medicaid program, a method by which an individual establishes Medicaid eligibility by reducing gross income through incurring medical expenses until net income (after medical expenses) meets Medicaid financial requirements.

Spiritual Practice: Spiritual discipline (often including spiritual exercises) is the regular or full-time performance of actions and activities undertaken for the purpose of inducing spiritual experiences and cultivating spiritual development.

Stress: A state of mental or emotional strain or tension resulting from adverse or very demanding circumstances.

Supplemental Security Income (SSI): A federal program that pays monthly financial assistance to people in need who are 65 or older and to people in need at any age who are blind or disabled. The purpose of the program is to provide sufficient resources so the person can have a basic monthly income. Eligibility is based on income and assets.

Support Group: A formal gathering of persons sharing common interests and issues. The participants and facilitators share information and mutual support, and often exchange coping skills with one another.

Surrogate: A substitute who makes decisions for someone who is no longer capable of making decisions for him/herself. The surrogate may be appointed as guardian or conservator by a court or identified when the person is declared incompetent through a power of attorney process.

Team: A group of people which may consist of family members, friends, church and community members who support the caregiver by assisting with the care of the care recipient.

Therapy: A treatment or intervention intended to change an outcome or course of disease.

Third-Party Payment: Payment for care that is made by someone other than the patient or his/her family (for example, Medicare or a private insurance company).

UTI—Urinary Tract Infection: An infection in any part of the urinary system such as kidneys, bladder and urethra. Most infections involve the lower urinary tract, the bladder and the urethra. Common among seniors, if untreated it may cause altered mental status and other serious complications.

Vital Signs: Temperature, pulse, respiration, and blood pressure.

Will: A written document which designates how property will be distributed after death. The will can be drafted with or without the assistance of an attorney.

Resources

Recommended Reading

The Bible
The American Book of Living and Dying, Richard Groves
and Henriette Anne Klauser
Caregiving for the Genius, Jane Barton
Creative Ideas, Ernest Holmes
Elder Rage, Jacqueline Marcell
Final Gifts, Maggie Callanan and Patricia Kelley
**How to Take Care of Old People Without Losing Your
Marbles,** Suzanne Asaff Blankenship
I Choose Me, Cynthia James
Jesus Calling, Sarah Young
On Death and Dying, Elizabeth Kubler Ross
Prayers that Avail Much, Germaine Copeland
**Resilience: The Science of Mastering Life's Greatest
Challenges**, Southwick and Charney
This Thing Called You, Ernest Holmes
The Last Lecture, Randy Pausch

Online Resources

AARP – Aarp.org
Adult Protective Services – Google for your local office
Alzheimer's Association – Alz.org
American Cancer Society – Cancer.org
American Psychological Association – Apa.org

Caregiver Action – CaregiverAction.org
Caregiver's Guardian – TcgCares.com
Caregiver's Veterans Administration – Caregiver.Va.org
Caring Bridge – CaringBridge.org
Family Caregiver Alliance – CareGiver.org
Griefshare – GriefShare.org
Healthcare – Healthcare.gov
Hospice Foundation of America – HospiceFoundation.org
Lotsa Helping Hands – LotsaHelpingHands.com
Medicare – Medicare.gov
National Institute on Aging – Nia.Nih.gov
Social Security Administration – Ssa.gov
Society of Certified Senior Advisors – Csa.us
Veterans Administration – Va.gov

Acknowledgments

To each of The Caregiver's Guardian clients, you were courageous in allowing me to contribute to your lives. Thank you for the honor of serving you and your families. Thank you for the lessons taught and for allowing me to share those lessons with others.

To my husband, Kevin, you are the greatest family caregiver I know. First with Mom, you were excellent in her care, and then with your parents, you left nothing to be desired. Though you didn't fully understand why I had to do this job or write this book, your love and support are invaluable and greatly appreciated. I love you more.

To my son, Rodrick Sean Freeman, your journey, your trials and your tests as you embarked upon writing your first book have been instrumental in inspiring me to move forward with this project. Continue your process in the manner you see fit and know that your story should and must be told. Your supporters are counting on you and so am I.

To my dad, Herman Roberts Jr., your faith in the Almighty has sustained me and lifted me when I didn't know where or how to turn. Thank you for always believing in me.

To Sharon Knox, my second mom, how grateful I am that you chose me as a daughter, mentee and confidante. Your support means the world to me.

To Cynthia James, my coach and mentor, your belief in me has been unwavering, and the bar you set in leading by example is higher than I imagined, but a call that I'm willing to answer.

To What Will Set You Free Freedom Coaches, this group of amazing coaches has been a tremendous support to me. You each exude excellence, dedication and commitment to your work that I gather tremendous strength from and seek to embody.

To The Sisters' Enterprise Master Mind Group, because of you, I met the challenge raised last year and I committed to completing this book. To Lisa Givens, Michelle Adams, Natasha Nelson, Larynda Jackson, Michelle Davis, Cherrelyn Napue and Kandice Porter, I extend my utmost appreciation.

To my team of initial reviewers: Sharon Knox, Cassandra Thames, Ellie T. Hough, Lisa Givens, Michelle Adams, Michelle Davis, Lynda King, Sam Trenke, Earl Wright, Jack Purnell, Althea Bruce, Roz Cary and Lori Goodwine, there are no words sufficient to express the depth of my gratitude to each of you for your candor, your encouragement and support. You gave me what I needed to move forward with this project. I am grateful to each of you.

To my mother's children: Demetrice, Earl and Anya, Derrell and Tina, Dexter and Ketrenna, Dwight and Robin, together we travelled the caregiving journey, loving and honoring Mom, hearing her voice as she said, "Y'all look out for each other. I won't always be here. Love conquers all."

To my sister/daughter, Larynda Jackson, I was blessed with nieces who are like daughters to me, but in you I found a sister, a friend and a daughter. Thank you for your integrity and the truth that you walk in. Thank you for allowing God's grace to flow through you.

To Nichelle Stiggers, Lutheran Family Services and The African American Caregiver's Support Group—yours is the best support group ever! Nichelle, thank you for your encouragement to launch TCG and the support you've provided me over the years. I have always admired, valued and appreciated you. Thank you for your presence in my life.

To Easter Seals and Stroke Survivor's Program—Donna and Jeff you are amazing *Anam Caras*. Your love, dedication and commitment are admirable. Thank you for being great examples and for being the extraordinary professionals you are. You both make me want to be better.

To the Boulder Briarpatch Book Club, you are the best group of intellectuals, free thinkers and forward thinking people I could ever hope to encounter.

To the Cornish family, the Roberts family and the St. Cyr clan, I love you all and appreciate the experiences shared, the love, joy and lessons that only a family can teach.

To my editors, John Maling, you were the male voice that I yearned to hear. You got me started and pointed me in the right direction. Cynthia Schoen, you were the answer to a prayer, the head chef, guardian and midwife that I needed to make this book the gift it is intended to be. Your prodding, pushing and teaching every step of the way helped create what I trust will be an encouragement to caregivers and their supporters for years to come. Thank you for the gift of you.

To Liana Moisescu, book cover designer, thank you for grasping the vision and creating a great cover.

To Ronnie Moore, interior designer, with gratitude and tremendous appreciation.

To the Author U community and Judith Briles, The Book Shepherd for teaching and providing a wealth of needed information to this new author.

To Lori Goodwine, PR Director and CIM Marketing Partners, thanking you in advance for all of the work that you are going to do to promote this book.

To all of my Spiritual Fathers, Mothers, Pastors, Counselors, Teachers who have supported me throughout the years. A special thanks to Apostle Phil Smith and my church home, Colorado Christian Fellowship. The following churches and leadership have had a profound impact on my life during my caregiving journey: For His Glory Christian Fellowship, Mile Hi Church, Den CO, Antioch Progressive Church, Sac CA, Christ Our Redeemer Church Irvine, CA and Greater St. Stephen Full Gospel, New Orleans, LA where my dad is Father of the Church.

To Mom Myra Bennett for the many pots of gumbo you've made and assisted me with. For your willingness to allow me to videotape you, for sharing your recipe, your techniques and your love, I'm so very grateful.

In Memoriam

At the time of the second printing of this book my cousin, Corneila Hill, caregiver extraordinaire, passed away at the age of 58. She spent the last decade of her life caring for her mother, and taking care of her family. The important message of "self care" first, is resonating loudly and firmly in Corneilia's memory.

About the Author

Nadine Roberts Cornish served as a devoted caregiver for her mother for 15 years. She had a 15-year background in Public Health Social Marketing Campaigns prior to her mother being diagnosed with a pituitary brain tumor.

Nadine founded The Caregiver's Guardian, LLC (TCG) in 2009, one year following her mother's death. A fierce advocate, researcher and champion for her mother, Nadine realized that not everyone had the resources or the skill set to do the same for their loved ones. Through TCG, she and her team of professionals have provided Care Management, Consulting and Caregiver Coaching services to assist family caregivers around the country in all facets of the caregiving journey.

A riveting and transformative speaker, trainer and educator, Nadine shares the lessons she learned through her personal journey and her travels with the family caregivers she has been blessed to serve. She uncovered resilience within herself and nurtures it in every caregiver she assists.

Nadine is a Certified Senior Advisor (CSA), and has earned a Professional Advancement Certification in Gerontology from the University of Colorado Gerontology Center. She is a Freedom Coach and Elite Life Coach.

How to Work with Nadine

Nadine works with clients nationally and throughout the Denver area. She coaches caregivers and their supporters with patience, encouragement and laughter via online video conferencing. She assists clients in every stage of the caregiving journey, including after the loss of a loved one.

In conjunction with her book, Nadine has launched a national movement called "Care-ocity." She is mobilizing businesses, organizations and churches to support caregivers and has developed a curriculum for full day and half day sessions. Nadine excels as a passionate and dynamic speaker. Contact her today!

Nadine Roberts Cornish, CSA
The Caregiver's Guardian, LLC
Certified Senior Advisor
Freedom and Elite Life Coach
303.394.1963
TearsInMyGumbo@gmail.com
TearsInMyGumbo.com
LinkedIn.com/In/NadineRobertsCornish-8590105
Facebook: @TearsInMyGumbo

Questions to Ponder

Rosalyn Carter said it best. There are only four kinds of people in this world: those who are caregivers, those who have been a caregiver, those who will be a caregiver and those who will need a caregiver.

Whether you choose to face it now or later, the reality is most of us will encounter the responsibility of caregiving sooner or later in life.

I invite you to ponder the questions on the next page. After taking time to give the questions some serious thought, I invite you to journal. Write about your thoughts and ideas pertaining to the questions asked. Write about how you feel and whether this topic is difficult for you. Hopefully, after reading this book, it will be a lot easier.

If you choose not to respond to any of the questions, that's fine. Take the time to simply write your thoughts. If you're a caregiver, then please start the process of writing, telling your own story. There is great value in capturing your thoughts and feelings through writing.

Questions for Support Group or Book Club

How do you view caregiving now and how did you view caregiving prior to reading this book?

Do you view caregiving as a burden, a responsibility or an honor? Why and what shaped your ideas?

Is caregiving something that you envision yourself doing should the need arise?

Are your affairs in order?

Is being cared for long term in your home a viable option?

Who might you have to take care of?

Who would you want in charge of your care?

Parents or Family Members in Need of Care?

Have you discussed your parents' wishes with them?

Are you comfortable supporting them as they have requested?

What stage of life are your parents in?

Do they have a chronic illness?

What plans are in place for their future care?

What role will you play in their future care?

Do you need a professional to assist you in planning their care?

For the Caregiver

What phase of conscious caregiving are you in?

What feelings are you experiencing?

What ingredients do you have on hand and what ingredients do you need?

Who have you enrolled to assist you on your caregiving journey? Who do you need to add to the mix to prepare a greater meal of care?

Have you developed a spiritual practice to help you maintain your spiritual and emotional wellbeing?

What outside resources could help you develop the expertise you need?

What About You?

What long term care plans do you have in place should you need to be cared for?

As your need for caregiving increases, will you want to continue living in your community or will you need to move in order to be closer to your loved ones?

How will you pay for long term care should the need arise? Review your long term care policy and make notes on what its terms, conditions and payments are.

Have you discussed your wishes with your adult children or designated person if you don't have children?

What are your wishes for how and where you'd like to live should you no longer be able to live alone?

Is there a family member that you would like to live with? If so, have you discussed your preference with them and all relevant family members? Have you placed it in writing?

What are your wishes for medical care during end of life? What are your preferences for your funeral and burial arrangements? Are these preferences included in your will and trust?

Journal your story, your wishes and your thoughts about caregiving.

Coming Soon

More of the *In My Gumbo* Series:

Prayers In My Gumbo

and

Joy In My Gumbo